COOK YOUR young

Improve Your Skin & Hair, Sleep Better,
Look & Feel Younger with 100 Easy Recipes

ELIZABETH PEYTON-JONES

photography by Yuki Sugiura

QUADRILLE

‘It's only when you understand that what you eat is life changing, that you can change your life.’

Introduction

This is a book to help you cook and eat more youthfully. It's a kind of DIY youthing manual, full of practical and easy ways to rejuvenate your brain, body, and immune system as well as any other bits you think might need some attention … The source of youthing power lies in your kitchen!

Just before I started writing this book, a journalist asked me, "Is food powerful?" A simple question, you'd think, but it stopped me in my tracks. I had never myself expressed it that way before. Powerful is a strong word, especially for something that we use/eat/cook with three times a day. It got me thinking. Can food really be described in that extraordinary way?

After not too much reflection, I concluded (you knew it!) that food is full of power. Phytochemical power, vitamins, minerals, protein, amino acids, enzymes, essential fatty acids, flavonoids, antioxidants, and a load of other nutritional nuggets … It produces energy and repairs your body. In extreme cases, it can kill you. It can also be the antidote. It contains almost everything you need to survive. Powerful? You bet.

Yet … today much of our food comes in boxes and packages from grocery stores. And, in a subtle way, that undermines our understanding of its intrinsic power. I often see people who don't realize that food is a life form that contributes to their own life form. They don't grasp that what they eat might be making them healthy and feel youthful, powerful, vibrant, and strong. Or unhealthy, old, angry, insipid, self-conscious, and dull. (And it can, let me assure you.)

This book is called *Cook Yourself Young: Harnessing the Power of Food* because it seemed genuinely important to me to reacquaint people with that fundamental food-body-power connection. If you want to feel fresh, awake, vibrant, youthful, inspired, and ready for new adventures, then look at what you eat. If you want to have clear, glowing skin, sparkling eyes, a lean physique, glossy hair, nails, and a body that works seamlessly well, as well as stave off colds, flus, and other bacterial illnesses, then your diet is fundamental.

That's the theory. Here's the application. Within these pages I want to:

★ Take healthy, youthing foods mainstream so they become your "new normal"
★ Help you understand what your body does with food, so you can feed it better
★ Give you hundreds of ideas, recipes, and suggestions so you can start cooking and eating youthfully right here, right now (and ditch addictive foods while you're at it)

Simple? You bet. OK, there are seven gentle principles to use as guidelines along the way (see pages 8 to 17) but you don't have to follow them slavishly; just let them inform your cooking, eating, and thinking around food. And there are four real-life studies of my clients, each of which shows how adopting a youthing lifestyle and eating plan can revolutionize the way you look, feel, and think.

I don't explore exercise or the power of the mind in this book. But it is imperative that, for optimum health, daily exercise for both body and mind is taken as seriously as the food that is eaten. Good food will help quieten the mind and allow for contemplation, which in itself can be life changing.

Of course, I can't promise miracles. But I know from experience that when clients change what they eat, they start to feel better remarkably quickly (we're talking weeks rather than months). They get leaner without feeling deprived. Their niggling symptoms (headaches, bad skin, aching joints and muscles, fatigue, brain fog) disappear. They start to look healthy and bouncy; they become more energetic and upbeat. They fall sick less often and don't need antibiotics, because they throw off illness more easily. (That's great news, not least because we are all entering an antibiotic-resistant world in which we can no longer rely on antibiotics to fight our bodies' battles for us.) They start experimenting with imaginative, tasty, and superhealthy youthing dishes such as those in this book ... and start having fun around food.

As soon as they're off that antiyouthing roller coaster they start looking, feeling, and living a healthier, leaner, more balanced, and energized life.

And as well as helping you look great and feel fabulous, this way of eating feeds your immune system and is therefore the foundation to great health. By removing the allergenic foods that inflame it and the processed foods that disrupt it, your immune system will be able to react more quickly, fight more strongly, and repair more effectively. Your body will overcome bacterial infections more easily and your need for antibiotics will diminish. Eating this way will help boost immunity, so your body can fight infections with vigor and rejuvenate much more effectively.

Just think about how astonishing that is.

That's the power of food.

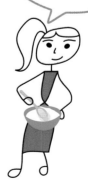

Start looking, feeling, and living a healthier, leaner, more balanced, and energized life.

BEFORE YOU START ...

You should know about five bodily processes and systems that can accelerate aging, but that you can overcome by choosing healthy, youthing foods.

Digestion: a well-functioning digestive system is the most important youthing tool. It's responsible for nutrient uptake, detox, immunity, and mood (as most of the body's serotonin is produced in the gut). You want this to run smoothly and to be problem-free ...

Inflammation: if this natural immune response becomes overreactive (as it tends to if you have food intolerances, a high-sugar diet, ongoing stress, exposure to chemical irritants ...) then you get chronic low-level inflammation in the body which is hugely aging. In fact, doctors have coined the word "inflamm-aging" to describe its toxic effects.

Acid and alkaline: the blood and intracellular fluid in your body work best when they are slightly alkaline. Eating too many acid foods (meat, dairy, processed foods, some grains, alcohol) can tilt them off balance, which means tissues are not repaired quickly, digestive disorders can arise, and—in the long term—an overacidic body can cause long-term damage and degenerative malfunctioning. You want to try and stay alkaline ...

Oxidation: oxygen is used by every cell in our body, but it is a bit of a loose cannon, always looking to combine with other molecules and, in the process, creating unstable "free radicals" that can cause cellular damage. Boosting the intake of antioxidants in your diet protects against this so-called oxidative stress, minimizing cellular degeneration and promoting youthing.

Immune system: your whole strength as a human—your ability to throw off colds, heal wounds, to repel, repair, and rejuvenate—is down to a well-functioning immune system. It works nonstop, flat-out to direct the epic "good vs bad" bacterial battle that is waging daily in and around your body. Eating nutrient-rich foods and minimizing the use of antibiotics, which kill off "friendly" bacteria along with the "unfriendly," is the key to keeping it in powerfully rejuvenative health.

Read on to start your new youthing life.

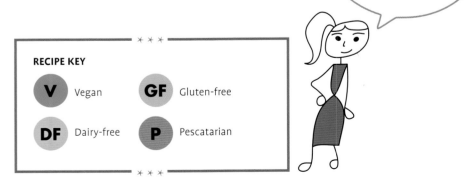

In 1700, people ate less than 11 lb [5 kg] of sugar a year. Three hundred years later, we're eating 154 lb [70 kg] a year.

* * *

RECIPE KEY

V Vegan **GF** Gluten-free

DF Dairy-free **P** Pescatarian

* * *

The New Normal

I see a lot of clients who have a terrible relationship with food. They treat certain foods as they'd treat an errant lover: one day they adore them and can't get enough; the next they want nothing more to do with them. They diet, then binge. They go to spas, lose 28 lb (13 kg) on a restrictive regime, then come home and turn into a round ball again. It's exhausting and debilitating. They're not getting the nutrients they need to stay young and vibrant. They have developed phobias around food that they can't answer one simple question: what can I eat?

This book is about finding the answer to that question. And then cooking it in the healthiest possible way to give your body the chance to look and feel all-round younger. It is a shortcut to rejuvenated skin, bright eyes, glossy hair, a leaner physique but also—crucially —to a new energy and zest that makes you look young to everyone you meet (and to your reflection in the mirror).

THE NEW NORMAL

So: what can we eat in a world bedeviled by too many (mostly bad) food choices? I'm on a mission to cut through all the nonsense and make healthy youthing foods mainstream: the new normal.

Let's face it, normal is not about dieting (diets, as we know, don't work). On the contrary. It is about choosing and cooking normal good-for-you youthing foods. But how do you achieve that sensible and happy state? I've had most success with clients when they start eating nutrient-dense foods "for health." This quickly makes them feel vibrant and energetic, debugs their system of niggles (the bad skin/hair/nails, headaches, joint pain, gut problems, low immunity, and extreme tiredness they didn't want to bother their doctor with), as well as inducing the delightful positive of looking five to 10 years younger within just a few months.

In Cook Yourself Young (CYY), I'll show you ways to cook for health and youthing using natural, nonprocessed foods that make us feel good and look even better, that satisfy us so that bingeing and blitzing and gimmicky diets are no longer part of our lives.

So let's keep it simple. Overleaf you'll find seven core principles that will help you create fabulous, tasty food using healthy ingredients that can decelerate the aging process and boost immunity. These principles will change your way of cooking and eating to make you look, feel, and live a healthier, leaner, more balanced, energized—and above all, younger—life. Keep them at the forefront of your mind and instinctively you'll choose the best youthing option for yourself and your loved ones and, this time, it will be easy and it will be for life.

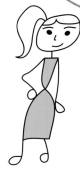

Keep to the principles but don't be slavish about them. Sometimes you just need to have fun around cooking and eating ...

THE FIRST PRINCIPLE: EAT THE NEW NORMAL; DROP ADDICTIVE FOODS

By addictive I mean processed foods, refined or hidden sugar, salt, and "bad" fats. These are dictionary-definition addictive, as they make your body crave more of them.

ADDICTIVE FOODS:

★ Processed foods made with refined flour and grains (white pasta, white rice, white bread, plus store-bought gunk such as pizzas, cookies, doughnuts, cakes, chips, and so on). Pretty much everything in a box or package

★ Anything with refined sugars (including sodas). Also pretty much everything in a box or package (notice a theme?)

★ Sodium chloride (salt): don't use it in cooking or sprinkle it on food; avoid high-salt smoked foods and ready meals

★ Processed meats such as salami, bacon, and sausages

★ Cow's dairy: with my delicious substitutes (see page 46), you'll barely notice the absence

★ "Low-fat" foods claiming to be organic or slimming. If it has more than a few ingredients, it is heavily processed

These induce cravings so you eat more of them more often, and they are nutrient-light and high-cal so you feel hungry while getting fatter. You get into an antiyouthing cycle of sluggishness and/or hyperactivity as the body is less able to process the toxin bombing from the overload of junk.

I think the slowly-slowly approach is harder. Why not just stop feeding the addiction? Give it up now: if you pack your diet with nutrient-rich new normal foods, your body will reacclimatize fast (and thank you for it).

HOW TO DROP ADDICTIVE FOODS?

There's a myth that it takes 21 days to kick a habit. I think that's tosh (and dangerous tosh, as you have one more reason to beat yourself up if you fail). Food addictions are tough to crack and my rule of thumb is to allow a week for each year of addiction. So, if you are 36 and have eaten lots of refined sugar since the age of 16, don't expect to be free of it until 20 weeks after you stop eating it. I know, that's longer than you'd expect, but be gentle on yourself …

SLOWLY-SLOWLY OR COLD TURKEY?

I think the slowly-slowly approach is harder. Why not just stop feeding the addiction? Give it up now: if you pack your diet with nutrient-rich new normal foods, your body will reacclimatize fast (and thank you for it). Note: some of my recipes contain maple syrup to add extra sweetness, but, if you are on a no-sugar diet, just leave it out.

THE NEW NORMAL: WHAT CAN I EAT?

I've given a list of 50 Stellar Youthing Foods (see pages 153 to 157). Add these to your diet at any opportunity you get. And stock up your New Normal pantry with:

★ Whole grains: amaranth, brown rice, millet, oats (try and sprout them if you can)

★ New normal flours: brown rice, buckwheat, hemp, millet, potato, quinoa, spelt, tapioca; and ground almonds, too

★ Fresh veg and fruit (as wide a range as you can)

★ Nuts, seeds, and my New Normal oils (see pages 10 to 11)

★ Beans, legumes, split peas (soak or sprout before use)

★ Herbs and spices (see pages 13 to 15)

★ Spirulina and chlorella (algae), wheatgrass, E3Live

★ Dried fruit in moderation: dates, apricots, raisins

★ Maple syrup or stevia (to be used in small doses!)

★ Himalayan/Celtic mineral salt: more minerals and saltier than table salt, so you use less. But, for youthing, cut all salt; use herbs, spices, and lemon juice instead

SHOULD I GO VEGAN, VEGETARIAN, OR RAW?

Going vegan is hip and you might think that cutting out dairy, meat, and eggs means you eat loads of healthy veg, beans, seeds, nuts, and fruit. But often vegans end up eating piles of pasta and other carbs and not much else. The result? Terrible skin (eczema, itchiness, dermatitis) and feeling low-energy, grumpy, and generally out of whack.

So, whether you're vegan, vegetarian, or raw, be creative so you get enough protein (nuts, seeds, beans, peas), minerals (especially iron, zinc, and selenium to prevent anemia), and vitamins (especially biotin and B-12 for skin, mental focus, and energy). Lots of my recipes are great for vegans and vegetarians: they'll boost mental and physical energy and give you all the nutrients you need for a youthing lifestyle.

WHAT IF YOU LAPSE?

Don't get spooked. Being normal is about being human, and humans have lapsed ever since the Garden of Eden. Allow for lapses. Some people restrict themselves all week and then, on Sunday, eat anything they want and, if this works for you (by which I mean you have no symptoms and are at the top of your game), then that's OK. In fact, it's much better than deciding to give up chocolate for ever and then wolfing down a bar the next day. Doing that leads to what I call "flabby willpower" and erodes your confidence in your own decision-making. Instead, I'd rather you took responsibility for your decisions (good or bad), positively decided to eat a bar of chocolate, and enjoyed every bite.

Take the long view. Once you start eating the New Normal, you'll lose your diet phobias and feel safe around food. You may have the odd blip. Forget it and move on.

THE SECOND PRINCIPLE: COOK YOUNGER

KNOW THIS: The way we cook food affects its nutritional and youthing benefits. I aim for high-nutrition cooking, which happens to be high-youthing cooking, too. The cooking process should retain maximum nutrients, antioxidants, and anti-inflammatories in all our food, to sustain us and keep us looking and feeling younger. So, how to do that?

HERE'S THE CYY WAY:

Dehydrating: One of the most youthing ways to cook. The food is in essence still raw and all the nutritional value has been kept. If you can eat 40 percent raw, including dehydrated foods, you are loading your plate with a varied array of nutrients and allowing your body to heal and rejuvenate on a daily basis.

Steaming: The best youthing option for most veg and fish. It allows food to retain goodness, as water-soluble vitamins don't leach away. Steaming veg with tough cellulose walls (spinach, carrots, and cruciferous leafy greens) makes nutrients more accessible. And it improves broccoli's youthing properties, as it helps produce carcinogen-kicking isothiocyanates in the body.

Steam-frying: My top way to cook youthing, tasty meals, as it brings the richness of frying with, typically, less than 1 tsp of oil (that tiny amount helps us absorb the essential fat-soluble vitamins A, D, E, and K). In terms of youthing, it allows for excellent nutrient retention.

HOW TO DO IT: Heat a heavy pan over medium heat until hot but not smoking. Add ½ tsp of avocado or coconut oil and swirl to coat. Add 4 to 6 Tbsp [60 to 90 ml] water, wait until it bubbles, then add the food. Cook as normal.

Slow cooking: Low-cost cooking in a slow cooker (or "crock-pot") gives high-energy, youthing results, because:

★ You don't need to add any oil

★ You won't get exposed to AGEs (advanced glycation end products), toxins that come from cooking meat at high temperatures. AGEs destroy collagen, so are aging for skin

★ Some nutrients are lost, but fewer than through boiling. (You can blanch vegetables to minimize enzyme loss before adding to the pot. But that adds an extra layer of faff ...)

★ Soups, stews, and curries become tender and tasty, if you whack in aromatic onions, garlic, spices, and dried herbs

WHAT YOU NEED: An electric slow cooker. These aren't expensive; you can get a 3-qt [3.5-L] version for around $20.

WHAT TO COOK: Fish, veg, grains.

NOTE: Don't cook dried beans in a slow cooker. They need to be boiled to neutralize toxins that can make you ill.

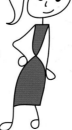

Instead of salt, squeeze lemon juice over the food you're steaming to intensify flavor.

NOT SO HOT

I'm not keen on broiling and barbecuing meat, boiling, microwaving, or deep-fat frying. Here's why:

Broiling and barbecuing meat: Charring or broiling meat or fish to give that caramelized taste produces inflammatory, collagen-destroying, and antiyouthing AGEs (see page 9). Cooking proteins at high temperatures also produces chemicals called HCAs and PAHs that can cause inflammation, speed cell damage, and increase the risk of chronic degenerative diseases including cancer. Both are listed on the US government National Institutes of Health's list of official cancer-causing agents.

Boiling: You may as well wash your nutrients down the sink. Cooking veg in lots of water at high temperatures leaches water-soluble vitamins and around 60 percent of mineral content. If the water turns a dark color, you are waving the antioxidants goodbye. Research shows that only artichokes and carrots seem to emerge unscathed from boiling.

HOWEVER: You do need to boil dried beans, to deactivate toxins that can make you ill.

Microwaving: I don't have a good thing to say about this. It's too easy to use the "wrong" container (which leaches chemicals into food), or to nuke veggies so they emerge as a tasteless, nutrient-light mush. As for youthing, I am convinced that microwaving changes food's structure and creates a negative impact on the body and, though we're years away from proving this, I don't want to take the risk.

Steaming veggies is easier and can help retain more nutrients. Take broccoli and other cruciform veg, for example: they contain a cancer-fighter called sulforaphane that is enhanced by steaming and depleted by microwaving. 'Nuff said.

Deep-fat frying: Just don't go there.

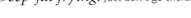

Avoid chemically-treated fats such as margarine or "healthy" spreads. They will do you no youthing good at all.

Poaching: Less nutrient-slaying than boiling, this is cooking for a short time in water just below boiling point. It's good for eggs, fish, and some fruits, but not for vegetables.

Roasting: I like to roast starchy veg such as potatoes, sweet potatoes, turnips, rutabagas, and beets as well as onions, garlic, carrots, and eggplants at a low temperature. You don't need fat, but it is delicious to sprinkle rosemary or thyme over veg for extra flavor. Add a drizzle of oil of your choice after the roasting has finished, to give that creamy taste.

Eat, drink broth: Remember that vegetable water your mom used to make gravy with? It's the water left over from steaming or poaching veg. Save it and use it as you would stock. Add it to risottos, stews, curries, hotchpotches, or when steam-frying; it's nutrient-rich, low-cal, and gives great flavor. Sometimes I even drink it cold in the morning as a youthing antidote to any food or drink excesses of the night before. Try it before you say ugh …

GET THE FATS RIGHT

The good fat/bad fat debate rages on, so for sanity's sake I like to keep it simple. For cooking, I use coconut oil or avocado oil. For drizzling, dipping, and so on, I add hemp, olive, and pumpkin seed oils. With these five, you have all the taste, nutrients, and youthing benefits you want.

As you know, fats are vital for our bodies to work properly, for healthy skin, for the proper functioning of cells, brain, and liver, and to process the fat-soluble vitamins A, D, E, and K. Counterintuitively, good fats even help weight loss: they make us feel satisfied so we eat less, but they also burn as energy rather than being stored in fat cells.

When you're buying oils, go for first cold-pressed extra-virgin, as these have not been degraded by heat in the extraction process. Choose oils in dark bottles and store in a cool, dark place (not near the cooker).

There is some evidence that microwaving removes nutrients. Take cruciform veg, for example: they contain cancer-fighting sulforaphane that is enhanced by steaming and depleted by microwaving.

Avocado oil: Use for cooking. It has a high smoke point (so won't degrade when heated, the chemical outcome of which causes inflammation). It's high in heart-healthy monounsaturated fats and omega-3 fatty acids, contains a heap of vitamins and minerals, plus protein. It helps with processing other nutrients, especially youthing carotenoids, can reduce blood pressure, is anti-inflammatory, and good for skin. A great multitasking oil.

GO CYY: The rich flavor gives dense creaminess to soups, smoothies, or mash. It's also delicious on salads and grains.

Coconut oil: This contains short- and medium-chain triglycerides, the same as those found in animal fats. The liver burns these as energy so, despite it being highly calorific, it can actually help with weight loss. It may help reduce blood cholesterol, too. I love the flavor and aroma.

GO CYY: Use in baking, curries, and high-heat cooking.

Hemp oil: This won't get you high, even though it's extracted from cannabis seeds! I love the nutty taste, and the great youthing benefits. It has a good balance of omega-3 to omega-6, contains essential fatty acids and some polyunsaturated fatty acids vital for youthful skin and joints, strong immunity, heart health, brain function, and mood. It's high in antioxidants, a good plant protein source (comparable to meat, fish, and eggs) and contains a natural dose of calcium, magnesium, potassium, and iron.

GO CYY: Don't cook with it (it has a low smoke point), but it's tasty drizzled on pasta and quinoa before serving. Add 1 tsp to thicken smoothies and make them more nutritious. Its nuttiness complements oily fish or it makes a tasty salad dressing with lemon.

> Have a couple of nuts when you snack on fruit; the protein prevents a sugar high and makes you feel less hungry later.

Olive oil: You'll be aware of its health and youthing benefits (it helps reduce inflammation, cholesterol levels, protect against diabetes and heart disease, and may help break down stored fat to encourage weight loss). Just don't cook with it (fry, broil, or roast) at high temperatures as it becomes unstable and can cause inflammation.

GO CYY: Drizzle over pasta, quinoa, or rice dishes, or use in salad dressings, mash, dips, add 1 tsp to smoothies …

Pumpkin seed oil: I love the deep green color and strong, earthy taste. It is full of zinc, fabulous for the immune system, skin, and bones. It helps regulate insulin and is good for sperm production. Not to be sniffed at! The sleep hormone tryptophan rates high in this oil: take some with a piece of fruit, for serotonin and melatonin to help sleep.

GO CYY: Though it has a high smoke point, heat destroys the flavor, so drizzle on baked potato or use in dressings.

Rice bran oil: I want to sneak in the very underrated and little used rice bran oil, derived from the germ and inner husk of the rice plant. The oil is a much lighter color than olive oil and looks insipid, but has a nutty taste. It has the added benefit of two unusual compounds: an antioxidant called gamma-oryzanol, which blocks the absorption of cholesterol into the body and tocotrienols which are a group of related fat-soluble compounds that easily convert to vitamin E, giving great skin and hair.

GO CYY: The reason I wanted you to know about this oil is that it has a very high smoke point, so is great for those very occasional dinners where frying, sautéeing, or baking is involved!

USING NUTS

★ If you're eating handfuls of nuts, soak overnight first. It rinses off tannins, making them taste better. It also kicks off sprouting, that activates enzymes to make nuts more nutritious and easier to digest. They can be dehydrated after being soaked for adding to salads, sprinkling in soups, or just for snacks

★ Store nuts in the refrigerator and throw them away at the first sign they're off. All high-fat foods can turn rancid

---

WHAT MAKES NUTS SO GREAT ...

Nuts are of course vegan, lactose-, gluten-, and wheat-free. But why are they so great for youthing? Five reasons:

1 Think about what a nut is: it's the egg of the plant world. It contains all the nutrients and genetic instructions to produce life. This means nuts contain protein and youthing phytonutrients a-go-go, from beautifying vitamin E to the free radical and cancer-fighter ellagic acid.

2 Specifically, they help with detoxifying, immune strength, and wound healing, protect against type-2 diabetes, and have a positive effect on blood vessels, cholesterol, and heart health. If you substitute nuts for meat and dairy, studies show a 45 percent reduction in heart disease risk.

3 Nuts are good deliverers of omega-3 and other healthy fats. These feed the cells, brain, muscles, joints, and skin, allow a speedy hormone messenger service to flow between cells, and help reduce inflammation.

4 Eat widely for a range of flavors and benefits: almonds, Brazils, cashews, coconuts, hazelnuts, macadamias, pecans, pine nuts, pistachios, and walnuts all have totally different tastes and slightly varying nutrient profiles. For example, eating a couple of Brazils a day is thought to decelerate the arrival of gray hair and reduce allergies and inflammation. Eating copper-rich hazelnuts neutralizes free radicals, while pistachios contain an anti-inflammatory that alleviates dermatitis and strengthens skin.

5 They don't make you fat. Although nuts are high in fat, what's remarkable is that people who eat them tend to be slimmer and therefore look and feel more youthful. This may be because the good fats they contain make you feel fuller and less likely to go on mad sugar binges.

THE THIRD PRINCIPLE: GO NUTS!

To practice successful youthing for life, you need to switch from being a predominantly dairy eater to being a nut eater (unless you are among the one percent of the population with a nut allergy, in which case skip this). It's part of your mission to become plant-powered! You'll notice that many of the recipes in this book use nuts (as milk, as flour, in smoothies, and desserts). That's because nuts offer major youthing bonuses and can, with a little expertise, be easily substituted for every kind of dairy. Let's give it a go.

Nut milk: An easy swap. Instead of cow's milk, use nut or seed milk. Make your own instead of buying processed long-life nut milks, it takes just five minutes (see page 46). DIY nut milk is more delicious and nutritious and wonderful for skin, hair, and nails (it's the vitamin E and omega-3s). Nut milks come in totally different flavors depending on the nut. If you are allergic to nuts try making rice milk, buckwheat milk, or pumpkin and sunflower seed milk. You make it in the same way.

GO CYY: Pour on cereals, use in smoothies, ice creams, add to hot drinks, use in baking. Or drink it fresh.

Nut yogurt: You can make yogurt from nut milk, using a probiotic yogurt starter (from health food or kitchen stores) and your nut milk of choice. Your body gets the same amount of good gut bacteria as from dairy yogurt.

Nut butters: These are *soooo* easy to make, try my Almond butter (see page 82). Nut butters have more taste and texture than dairy butter, so you can't substitute them for butter when baking; I tend to use coconut oil or butter in baking (see pages 134 to 152).

Nut cheese: Try my creamy nut cheeses (see page 81). They are delicious and work as toppings on bakes or sprinkled on soups. They are best with intense flavor bursts from herbs and spices: try garlic, chile, chives, cumin, whatever makes your taste buds come alive.

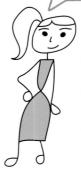

At the very end of slow cooking, add a handful of just-cut herbs to give a fresh flavor burst.

THE FOURTH PRINCIPLE: GET THERAPY WITH HEALING HERBS AND SPICES

I'm always amazed by how timid we are about using herbs in the Western world. Adding 1 tsp of dried oregano here or a garnish of parsley leaves there just doesn't hack it in the youthing stakes. One of my missions is to herb up the nation (that's "beef up" for plant fans) and encourage you to whack huge bundles of herbs and plenty of spices into your dishes, so you can take advantage of their fabulous rejuvenating effects.

Herbs and spices pack an industrial-size nutrient punch: they are intensely powerful. Many pharmaceutical drugs are based on the bioactive constituents of these plants; in fact, 40 percent of anticancer drugs developed between 1940 and 2002 were derived from natural plant products. We like herbs for their intense flavors and these come from the volatile oils that also provide an incredible range of therapeutic and youthing benefits (see right for a few!).

Generally speaking, herbs are antioxidant, alkalizing, and anti-inflammatory. They are free-radical fighters, immune-boosters, and detox helpers. They do pretty much all the youthing you need: strengthen cells, joints, muscles, veins, blood, and organs; make eyes, hair, and nails shine; heal skin; make you happy. Youthing therapy.

Please use herbs prolifically. Chuck handfuls of parsley, cilantro, dill, and other leafy herbs into casseroles minutes before serving. Use herbs as vegetables: make soups with them, or eat them raw in salads. Add exotic spices to dishes and smoothies to bring flavor fabulousness and nutrient intensity to your diet. Eat lots of different kinds (not just from the list below). For example, if you enjoy foraging, pick young nettle tops in late spring when they are sweetest (wear long gloves!) for soup or pesto, or add dandelion leaves to salads. Both these herbs (some call them weeds) are high in chlorophyll and rejuvenating minerals and vitamins. In other words, see herbs as a food, not a decoration. A major player, not a bit part. Your body will thank you for it.

If you use dried herbs or spices, buy organic if you can as the nutrients won't have been blitzed by irradiation ...

NOTE: If you use dried herbs or spices, buy organic varieties if you can as, that way, their nutrients won't have been blitzed by irradiation ...

10 HERBS AND SPICES YOU CAN'T LIVE WITHOUT

Garlic and turmeric are in my top five youthing foods for their hormone-balancing, anti-inflammatory properties. Mint and nutmeg are up there, too (see page 155). As for the 10 others I have highlighted here, I really can't cook or live youthfully without them ...

Basil: Awesomely flavorful and superyouthing for the digestion (killing bugs, worms, and viruses), cancer-fighting, and with flavonoids that help protect cell structure and function. High in vitamin K, which strengthens bones.

GO CYY: Use in pesto, salads, soups (especially tomato), stir-fries, or as basil tea (delicious, honestly). The oils are volatile, so add to food at the end of the cooking process. I like a bit of chopped basil in lemon ice pops, too.

Cinnamon: I use this liberally as it reduces blood sugar levels; when eaten with sweet foods it helps stabilize sugar spikes. It's also anti-inflammatory, kills bacteria and fungi so is fantastic for the gut, and is cholesterol reducing; a total must-have in the youthing larder.

GO CYY: Add to sweet foods—desserts, cakes, breads, smoothies—or eat with fruit to minimize sugar rushes. Fantastic in Indian dishes and curries, too.

Cilantro/ coriander: Leaves or seeds. This power-packed anti-inflammatory can reduce blood sugar and cholesterol and help digest fats. It's used to help with diabetes and to lessen anxiety, so it's a youthing all-rounder ...

GO CYY: Add ground seeds to meat, lentil, and grain dishes; it's a mainstay in Indian curry spice mixes. Cilantro leaves are delicious in salads, are the taste backbone of guacamole, and make a great alternative for basil in pesto.

Calling all students: before you go into an exam, take a deep inhalation of rosemary. It can wake up the brain and improve memory. Put some dried rosemary in a small cloth and tie a string around it. Rub it into your palm to get the essential oils active, then sniff!

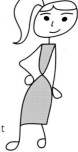

GO CYY: THREE WAYS TO STORE HERBS FOR WINTER

1 **Freeze them:** Good for herbs with a high water content, such as basil, chives, mint, parsley, and tarragon. Spread the dry leaves out on a baking sheet lined with parchment paper. Freeze. Next day, tip into freezer containers and store in the freezer. Their nutrients and flavor last for about three months.

2 **Ice cube them:** Mince dry herbs, and put into ice-cube trays so each hollow is one-third full. Cover with broth or water. Once frozen, store the cubes in freezer containers. Add two or three to casseroles.

3 **Dry them:** Good for herbs without much water content, such as dill, oregano, rosemary, or thyme. Place the leaves apart on a baking sheet lined with parchment paper. Place in the oven on its lowest setting, leaving the door ajar, for three to five hours until dried. Store in an airtight dark glass jar.

GO CYY: DIY TEA

If you're already adding fresh herbs and spices to your morning smoothies, then why not drink them as tea, too? You get intense youthing in a tisane. Here's how to make herb tea:

The leafy version (for one mug)
STEP 1: Put a handful of washed leaves (such as mint/basil/rosemary) in a glass teapot or bowl.
STEP 2: Pour over a big mugful of just-boiled water.
STEP 3: Leave for five minutes, then strain and drink.

The rooty version (for one mug)
STEP 1: Peel and chop a root (such as ginger/licorice/dandelion) to give ½ to 1 oz [15 to 30 g]. Put in a pan with 2 cups [500 ml] of water.
STEP 2: Bring to a boil; simmer for 10 minutes.
STEP 3: Strain, then drink.

Cumin: A good detoxer and youthing free-radical scavenger, cumin may also help with nutrient uptake as it stimulates the production of pancreatic enzymes. And it's thought to protect against cancer. It's also the secret ingredient in so many Middle Eastern dishes …

GO CYY: Buy as seeds or ground spice. I use it liberally in soups and rice, grain, and bean dishes. Sprinkle in home-made nut cheese (see page 81). Good in breads, Mixed seed crackers (see page 53), smoothies, and carrot cake.

Fennel: Whether vegetable bulb or seeds, this ticks a heap of youthing boxes. It's anti-inflammatory and extremely good for the digestive system because it is antifungal (so a candida-fighter), and antibacterial. It's also high in antioxidants, vitamins, and minerals.

GO CYY: Eat the bulb raw in salads, or you can barbecue and roast it, too. It's great with fish. Toss cooked fennel in lemon and oil and eat with zucchini "pasta" (see page 114). Or sprinkle seeds in smoothies and sauces.

Ginger: Soothing on the digestion, antinausea, and anti-inflammatory so good for joints. Studies have found ginger helpful with osteoarthritis, aching muscles, and musculoskeletal disorders and also in halting tumor growth.

GO CYY: Superversatile in sweet or savory foods and in smoothies. Great as a tea. Use root or ground ginger.

Lavender: A mood and sleep enhancer used to help with anxiety and depression and soothe the nervous system. It can ease headaches, too. The essential oil found in the flowers is what you need for youthing and you can dry the buds. Some people inhale the essential oil or use a lavender pillow, but I like to eat it, too.

GO CYY: Add dried lavender to meat dishes instead of oregano, sage, or thyme and use it to flavor cakes and baked goods, too. Drink lavender tea before bedtime.

Parsley: Whoppingly high in chlorophyll, vitamin C, folic acid, iron, and other minerals, with anti-inflammatory flavonoids which act as free-radical scavengers, this herb also has anticancer and blood sugar-reducing effects. Parsley is a youthing essential. Eat regularly!

GO CYY: Parsley can be used as you would salad greens,

in smoothies and tabbouleh, or add it to soups, pesto, casseroles, or stir-fries. Add the leaves near the end of cooking, to retain the nutritional value.

Rosemary: An antiaging multitasker containing powerful antioxidants and anti-inflammatories, which also works as a gentle liver detoxer. This herb also stimulates the immune system and helps to improve the digestion. Rosemary strengthens tiny blood vessels good for the skin and blood flow to the brain, which may be why it is called the herb of remembrance ...

GO CYY: This is my herb of choice with roasted veg, meat, and fish (it is traditionally used with meat because it helps in the production of bile which breaks down saturated fats). It's delicious in breads, crackers, and salads. Drink as tea or use to flavor nut milk.

Eating a 40 percent raw diet will alkalize you. I'm a fan of raw food, with some exceptions—the dreaded "raw" energy bars and processed "raw" foods—so avoid these! I mean foods as close to their natural state as possible.

Thyme: A great antioxidant that also (like rosemary) helps brain function and boosts immunity in the gut. One study showed it even slowed the effects of aging in animals. Its essential oil—thymol—is one of the main ingredients of commercial mouthwashes, because of its antiseptic qualities.

GO CYY: Thyme is a traditional ingredient in bouquets garnis and is delicious in soups, broths, casseroles, fish, meat, and egg dishes. Use the herb fresh if you can, when the thymol and other powerful flavonoids will be stronger.

THE FIFTH PRINCIPLE: WASH YOUR INSIDES EVERY DAY

Imagine your body as a washing machine. If it isn't regularly sluiced through with water and soap, grungy bits build up in odd places and it stops working properly. To avoid that happening to your insides, you need to put on a daily wash using water and some metaphorical "soap," followed by a nice cleansing rinse. It will get all your internal body systems working smoothly and at top-notch, and also build good bacteria in the gut. Here's how:

1 Drink 2 cups [500 ml] first thing: Preferably a whole lemon squeezed into warm water (you can add ginger, if you like), or a green juice. If you are feeling low in energy, juice a mix of beet, carrot, ginger, spinach, and lemon; about 1 cup [250 ml] of that will pep you right up.

I know when I am too acidic because I wake up feeling draggy. So I up my alkaline intake by making a green juice first thing and having spirulina and chlorella shots throughout the day.

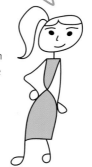

ONCE YOU GET A SPICE IN YOUR HOME, YOU HAVE IT FOREVER.
WOMEN NEVER THROW OUT SPICES.
THE EGYPTIANS WERE BURIED WITH THEIR SPICES.
I KNOW WHICH ONE I'M TAKING WITH ME WHEN I GO.

ERMA BOMBECK, JOURNALIST

PIMP MY WATER: WHAT'S IT DOING IN THERE?

1 builds: Body parts—cells, organs, muscles, joints, blood, lymph, digestive juices—are made of water.

2 lubricates lymph, digestive, and nervous systems.

3 transports nutrients and chemicals around the body (via the blood, spinal fluid, saliva, and so on).

4 regulates temperature via sweat and respiration.

5 detoxes by flushing waste out of the body.

WHAT IS HEALTHY WATER?

"Bottled drinking water" can come from any source, while those labeled "purified" or "vapor distilled" are processed tap water. Avoid.

Distilled water: drink with caution, though good for detoxing. It is boiled and condensed, which strips out contaminants and pulls toxins from your body (along with minerals).

"Natural mineral water": from natural springs, bottled at source. Normally alkaline, relatively pure, and with the right mix of minerals and trace elements.

"Spring water": from a natural underground source, mineral-rich, but may be chemically treated.

Drinking water: often contaminated by bacteria, drugs, heavy metals, and chlorine and with some minerals removed. But filtered drinking water is better than none: just make sure you get your minerals elsewhere.

2 Eat a small amount of fermented food (separately from other foods). Take a probiotic pill daily. If you think you have parasites or fungi take an antifungal (oregano, caprylic acid) and antiparasitic herbs (black walnut, wormwood, clove oil) to keep your gut robust and build immunity.

3 Drink regularly: If you can do a bit more internal rinsing, all to the good; I'd advise drinking 6½ cups [1.5 L] or even more each day. It can be water, herb or green teas, homemade juices … anything but caffeine- or sugar-rich drinks (no coffee, cola, soda, or energy drinks).

That's all there is to it! Do this every day and you can consider your body youthfully cleansed.

THE SIXTH PRINCIPLE: EAT 40 PERCENT RAW TO ALKALIZE, AND SPROUT YOUR PROTEIN

This principle is about quick and easy alkalizing. What's that? It's a pathway to optimum youthing. It is about keeping blood and intracellular fluids slightly alkaline, when they work best. Our bodies are great at doing this …

★ But sometimes because of bad diet, stress, and so on, our bodies become slightly acidic. To counteract this, minerals (especially calcium and magnesium) may be pulled from bones, weakening them. Acid wastes build up and have to be eliminated through the skin, liver, and colon, or they will be dumped in fatty tissue. An acidic body is an open arena for the development of inflammation and degenerative diseases

★ Instead of eating acid foods (meat, dairy, lots of grains), boost your diet with alkaline veg and seeds. Try for around 60 percent alkalizing to 40 percent acid-forming foods. Remember, fruit contains sugar so is essentially acidic. Eat it sparingly (no more than two servings a day). Check to see if you need to alkalize (see page 24)

YOU SAID EASY ALKALIZING?

Life's short and I like to keep it faff-free. So instead of studying food alkalinity charts before a meal, just do this:

Eat 40 percent of your food raw.

That's a salad for lunch, a green juice with breakfast, some Mixed seed crackers (see page 53), and a salsa during the day and you're done.

THE DAILY RAW

Raw food is intrinsically alkalizing because it is mostly veg, a bit of fruit, nuts, and seeds. (There are some exceptions—including the dreaded "raw" energy bars and processed "raw" foods—but avoid these!) I especially like to eat sprouts, as they are easier to digest than vegetables and have more nutrient density because they are packed full of protein, ready to make a plant. However, I'm not wedded to eating a high raw diet: some foods contain more nutrients when raw, others are better cooked. Yes, cooking can destroy the vitamins in some veg—vitamin C and folic acid are particularly vulnerable—but the losses are unlikely to affect your body's regenerative abilities. Instead, what I like about the 40 percent raw rule is:

★ Veg and fruit are generally very high in fiber, so great for gut health, which is central to the youthing process

★ No one has interfered between you and your raw food (especially if you buy organic). That means the foods are free from extra-loading with sugars and fats

★ Veg, fruit, nuts, and seeds are nutrient-dense, antioxidant, and anti-inflammatory; they tick our youthing boxes

★ Chewing on hard veg is a workout for your teeth and jaw muscles, helping to keep them healthy

★ Raw food boosts vitality, rejuvenates skin and joints, and keeps the immune system strong (and veg juice counts)

WHICH MEANS THAT:

★ Anyone, anywhere, can manage this

THE SEVENTH PRINCIPLE: YOUTH YOUR KITCHEN

You could spend weeks hunting down youthing, nontoxic cooking utensils that don't scratch, peel, chip, crack, or leach. But I've decided one simple rule cuts to the heart of the matter: do not cook with any utensil you would not like to chew on. Do you enjoy putting plastic or food wrap in your mouth? No, thought not ...

So don't use ...

★ Plastic, silicon, or PVC spatulas, cutting boards, bottles, storage containers, or plastic wrap. Think of it like this: The plastics they are made of will degrade over time and sooner or later you will be swallowing the chemicals they contain. These include nasties such as BPA (bisphenol A), shown to affect the nervous and immune systems in animals as well as linked to coronary heart disease and hormonal changes in humans

★ Aluminum and nonstick pans: Because many people believe they leach the chemicals they are made from or are coated with into the food you cook

Instead try ...

★ Nature-based utensils such as wooden spatulas and cutting boards (their oils also make them naturally antiseptic); ceramic or glass pots; breathable cheesecloth food covers; glass (not plastic) straws. All are cheap and easy to find. You can put plastic wrap over cheesecloth food covers to stop the food degrading, as it won't then touch the food

★ Use dishes made from glass and pans that are enamel-coated: they can be heated to high temperatures without any problems. Or use cast-iron or heavy stainless-steel pans, but not if they are chipped or scratched

YOUTHING GIZMOS YOU MIGHT LIKE

★ A juicer (masticating, centrifugal, fusion)

★ A mandolin, for fine veg slicing

★ A handheld blender (for soups)

★ A steamer (with two baskets)

★ A bristle veg-scrubbing brush

★ An electric slow cooker

★ A food processor (for chopping)

★ A dehydrator

Strip out the strip lighting in your pantry; it can heat the food inside. Cool food makes you younger!

I've decided one simple rule cuts to the heart of the matter: do not cook with any utensil you would not like to chew on. Do you enjoy putting plastic or food wrap in your mouth? No, thought not ...

Body Works

So: Your body works brilliantly without you paying any attention to it all your life ... until suddenly it doesn't. You wake up one morning and your skin looks tired; you have 21 annoying ailments (including stiff joints, flabby belly, indigestion, lack of energy); you're exhausted and can't find joy in life. And you're not sure how you got here.

A clue: Your body is a system, compiled of subsystems that interact in the most beautiful way. When one part of the ecosystem gets out of whack, it has a knock-on effect on another. The symptoms show up in strange places: who would think an intolerance to a food or chemical could be due to an overworked immune system?

To age youthfully, you have to pick up on those symptoms and do something about them. Quickly. Before your complex, interactive body starts to get overburdened. You have to find out what the symptoms mean.

In the interests of youthing, opposite is an outline of the most important nutrient-delivery and emission organs. I've concentrated on food and waste processors, those you need to look after to help your body live in the most youthful way possible.

* * *

CYY BREATHING
This is a breathing detox: do it twice a day, or more if you are feeling stressed or low in energy. It has a triple youthing effect: it's calming, it increases the involuntary muscle contractions in the gut (peristalsis) and also oxygenates the blood. This helps food to be broken down into its nutrient parts more efficiently and for these nutrients to be better distributed via the blood to all areas of the body. But be warned: This exercise can make you feel quite high, it's amazing what a bit of oxygen can do for the system!

This breathing process will take just a few minutes, and you can do it anywhere.

STEP 1 Let all the old breath out, exhaling slowly from your lungs.

STEP 2 Breathe in deeply through your nose (the gateway to the brain), count to 10 as you are breathing, being aware that you are filling up your belly rather than your lungs.

STEP 3 Hold your breath for a count of 10.

STEP 4 Exhale slowly from your mouth, counting to 10.

STEP 5 Inhale once more from your nose for 10 counts, hold for 10, then exhale for 10.

Repeat the breath five times more.

* * *

IMPORTANT YOUTHING ORGANS

SKIN (eliminative)
The largest organ and our first defense.
It also eliminates water-soluble toxins
via sweat. It's easy to notice when other
organs are blocked and your skin is left
to do the elimination: you get spots,
discoloration, dryness, or lines (though
it's not always that straightforward).

LUNGS (eliminative)
Some toxins leave the body via the lungs.
But when we don't breathe properly, this
"detox" is less effective. If your breathing
is shallow, you might notice shortness of
breath; aching chest muscles; shoulder
tension; even emotional upset. Try daily
CCY Breathing (see previous page).

STOMACH
A churning bag of acid, enzymes, and
mucus whose job is to make big bits
of food small, before they enter the
intestine. If it underperforms (low acid)
or overperforms (high acid) you know
about it from signs such as burping, gas,
bloating, acid reflux, ulcers, or heartburn.

LIVER (eliminative)
A multitasker in charge of removing
toxins; processing nutrients; making bile;
and building proteins, among other jobs.
It is the pit pony of the body, in need of
regular TLC. If it doesn't get it, symptoms
of dysfunction—and feelings of old age—
are likely to crop up.

KIDNEYS (eliminative)
These filter blood, removing waste. They
balance electrolytes and acidity, so cells
and fluids can function optimally. They
regulate blood pressure and production
of red blood cells. Healthy kidneys are
essential to youthing, to prevent swelling
and weight gain, and to excrete toxins.

GALL BLADDER
Where bile, an alkaline fluid, is stored.
When you eat, it releases bile to break
complex fats into essential fatty acids,
so their nutrients can be used. If it
underperforms you can get indigestion,
nausea, pale stools and—in extreme cases
—the severe pain of gall stones.

LYMPHATIC SYSTEM
This transports lymph, a fluid that helps
rid the body of waste. It is vital to keep
it clean and moving or glands in the
appendix, spleen, thymus, tonsils, and
groin can swell and toxicity will set in.
Skin brushing, deep breathing, regular
exercise, and plenty of fluids will help.

PANCREAS
This makes pancreatic juice, an alkaline
liquid that breaks down proteins,
fats, and carbs and is sluiced into the
intestine, where the enzymes get to
work. It also releases hormones that
regulate blood glucose, which is crucial
for youthing and to prevent diabetes.

DIGESTIVE TRACT (eliminative)
If the eliminative process is not
working properly, toxins can cause
inflammation and food intolerances.
People who eat too much meat
or not enough fiber can develop
pouches in the intestinal wall. Over
time, these become infected, in an
aging condition called diverticulitis.

THE INSIDE STORY

In my line of business you get a bit obsessed with the workings of the human digestive system. It's complex and does *amazing things*, such as process a chemical wonderland of fats, carbs, proteins, vitamins, and minerals on a minute-by-minute basis. Such as *get rid of unhelpful wastes and toxins*. And produce 90 percent of the body's feel-good serotonin hormone. And be home to more immune cells than the whole of the rest of your body. This is where the chemistry of life happens.

For good youthing, we need to get the *gut stuff* right. It is fundamental to nutrient absorption, hormonal integrity, alkalizing, detox, a robust immune system … the whole lot.

But clients often tell me they don't know the first thing about how the body turns the food it eats into the nutrients it needs. So, here's a brief guide to food's short (and not so sweet) journey through the processing factory that is our digestive system.

LUNCH AND BEYOND …

You're hungry. It's lunchtime, saliva is flowing, and you take a bite of your houmous salad sandwich. What happens next? Basically, five simple steps:

STEP 1 CHEW: Your jaws move and teeth bite, your tongue pushes food around, the *enzymes* in your saliva start the process of breaking down the carbs in your bread. After 10 to 40 chews (more is better for youthing!), the food is a soft pellet called a "bolus."

STEP 2 SWALLOW: The bolus slips into the food pipe (esophagus). Using 50 pairs of muscles and nerves, it takes a few seconds to be pushed down into your *stomach*.

STEP 3 LIQUIDIZE: The stomach is like a washing machine: a seething mix of muscle power, enzymes, and gastric acids that turn food into a soupy consistency called chyme, made from amino and fatty acids. Food starts to be *broken down* into nutrient parts in the stomach while the acid kills bacteria, too. Food stays in the stomach for up to four hours (protein takes longest to process, but veg juice can go through in 20 minutes), then heads to the small intestine.

STEP 4 ABSORB: This is the miracle part. In the first bit of the small intestine (called the duodenum), the *pancreas* releases enzyme-rich juices that further break down protein, as well as carbs and fats. The *liver* and *gall bladder* produce and release enzyme-rich bile, which helps the absorption of fats. Intestinal juices join the party. All are alkaline, so neutralize stomach acid. It takes chyme about four hours to pass through the 22-ft [6.7-m]-long small intestine, during which time specific nutrients (vitamins, minerals, glucose, fatty acids, amino acids) are grabbed by tiny, highly specialized "fingers" (called villi) and absorbed through the walls of the small intestine into the bloodstream. You are being fueled.

STEP 5 EXCRETE: What's left moves into the five-foot-long large intestine. Any remaining absorbable nutrients—especially vitamin K—are extracted through the walls of the large intestine; meanwhile digestive mucus and gut flora get mixed in. This waste is pushed down the intestines by muscular contractions (peristalsis) and eventually (24 to 72 hours later) comes out as feces.

There you have it

> Most people go to the bathroom perhaps once a day. I'd like you to eat more fiber-rich foods and go two to three times a day, so the bowels aren't sluggish or overburdened and you avoid bloating, indigestion, wind, bad breath, and IBS.

For good youthing, we need to get the gut stuff right. Digestion is fundamental to nutrient absorption, hormonal integrity, alkalizing, detox … the whole lot.

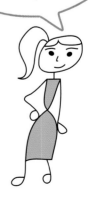

WHAT ARE ENZYMES?

Your body can't absorb that houmous sandwich per se, it has to break it down into individual nutrients first (that's amino acids, glucose, fatty acids, vitamins, and so on). Digestive enzymes make this happen. They are food processors that turn big food molecules into smaller food molecules so the body can use them. Each type of enzyme has a specific job:

★ Proteases break down proteins to produce amino acids
★ Lipases break down fats to produce fatty acids and cholesterol
★ Carbohydrases break down carbs to produce glucose or simple sugars
★ Lactases break down milk to produce lactose (milk sugar)

Enzymes are mostly produced in the pancreas and small intestine, but the salivary glands and stomach also make some more that kick off the breakdown of (respectively) carbs and proteins.

ENZYME POOR?

If your digestive enzymes aren't in great shape, you may notice some symptoms:
★ food allergies or intolerances
★ bloating and gas after eating
★ a stone-in-the-stomach feeling
★ undigested bits of food in your feces
★ floating or greasy-looking feces
★ poor wound healing

Boost production by eating enzyme-rich foods including raw veg, fruit, seeds, and nuts, especially pineapple, papaya, and sprouted foods. Juicing sprouted and raw foods ensures good enzyme activity. You can also buy digestive enzymes in supplement form from health food stores.

ANTIYOUTHING BUSTERS

★ When digestion and elimination are underperforming or weak, the body becomes *nutrient-deficient* and stressed; pretty soon you'll notice unexpected *early signs of aging*. These can range from lined skin, broken veins, and weight gain to low energy and immunity, stomach problems, inflamed joints, and brain fog. And then there's low mood, disturbed sleep, and "heat" issues (heartburn, acne, burning eyes, acid tummy ...).

To bust the *antiyouthers* and get back on track, see if you suffer from any of these symptoms and follow the *youthing* strategies below:

ANXIETY

★ Anxiety is antiyouthing: it overstresses the adrenal glands, exactly the wrong prescription for healthy cellular functioning. A whole range of symptoms can come with it: Tension headaches, backache, palpitations, breathlessness, dry mouth, dizziness, or stomach upsets. Changing your diet can help, by eliminating stimulants and smoothing out sugar and lactic acid levels in the blood.

GO CYY: Try cutting out caffeine, alcohol, and sugar. Beef up your intake of B vitamins, calcium, and magnesium by eating leafy green veg, beans, whole grains, seeds, sea vegetables, nuts, mushrooms, lentils, and oatmeal. Sing while making food!

RECIPES TO TRY: Avocado mousse wrapped in spinach; Thai fish curry; Banana bread (see pages 92, 111, and 49).

BRAIN FOG

★ Sometimes you get fuzzy thinking, poor concentration, or memory loss. That's brain fog.

GO CYY: Eat foods with vitamin D (the lack of which is linked to dementia: Oily fish or egg yolk. It gets harder to synthesize vitamin D from sun as you age, so you can take cod liver oil supplements or eat foods fortified in vitamin D (try juice or yogurt).

RECIPES TO TRY: Salmon and salsa "sandwiches" with quinoa; Scrambled egg breakfast muffins; vegetable juices (see pages 112, 38, and 41 to 46).

> *Food insensitivities and allergies can be a factor not just in celiac disease and other chronic digestive problems, but also in antiyouthing disorders such as depression, skin problems, joint pain, fatigue, and low immunity.*

EYES

★ Puffy bags under the eyes may be to do with edema (swelling), showing the kidneys need help.

GO CYY: Eat antioxidant-rich foods low in potassium and phosphorus (as these are hard for the kidney to process). These include all veg and fruit, especially those which are red or purple all the way through (red bell peppers, red cabbage, raspberries, blueberries). Eat fish and eggs for protein, avoid alcohol and salt. Drink cucumber juice.

RECIPES TO TRY: Vegetable juices; Gazpacho; Split pea dhal; Blackberry pastilles (see pages 41 to 46, 55, 115, and 138).

★ If your eyes are bloodshot, yellowish, or have dark brown shadows underneath, your liver needs support.

GO CYY: For a serious boost, give up alcohol and get foraging—eat nettles (soup or pesto), parsley, drink dandelion tea—also try milk thistle tea.

RECIPE TO TRY: Chia tabbouleh (see page 76). Or try making your own nettle pesto.

★ If your eyelashes or brows are thinning, it can show your metabolism has slowed, you're stressed, and your adrenal glands and thyroid need support.

GO CYY: Eat sea vegetables, seafood.

RECIPES TO TRY: Cod Provençal; Quinoa maki rolls (see pages 118 and 89).

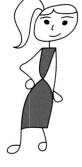

> If you want to see digestive enzymes at work, buy some capsules (from health food stores) and break open a couple into a bowl of oatmeal. Within 20 minutes, you'll notice the oatmeal starting to break down.

FATIGUE

★ An unnatural degree of tiredness is youth-sapping, you never have get up and go. If you sleep OK, instead look at your diet, as you may be adrenally stressed.

GO CYY: To support the adrenals, give up sugar, caffeine, alcohol, and refined carbs, they give a fast "false" energy that, in the long-run, wipes you out. To wake your body up, drink lemon juice with ginger in warm water or as a tea first thing in the morning; then have two alkalizing "dense green drinks" a day: juice up chlorella, barley grass,

---

ARE YOU ALLERGIC?

Food insensitivities and allergies can be a factor not just in celiac disease and other chronic digestive problems, but also in antiyouthing disorders such as depression, skin problems, joint pain, fatigue, and low immunity. The most common are to wheat, soy, dairy, nuts, shellfish, sugar, and alcohol, but some people are allergic to citrus fruits, fish, or even artichokes.

How do you know if you are allergic or intolerant to any foods? If you feel tired all the time, get a lot of respiratory sniffles, or feel generally under the weather, try an elimination diet; it can help pinpoint problem areas. Eat only hypoallergenic foods such as sweet potato, brown rice, broccoli, cabbage, zucchini, avocado, sea fish (nonfarmed), banana, apple, and pear for a week. Your symptoms might disappear by day five or six.

Now gradually reintroduce other foods (one every couple of days) to see if symptoms recur; that way you will know which foods cause you the problem.

ARE YOU INFLAMED?

Chronic inflammation happens when the body can't properly switch off its immune response. "Inflamm-aging" can damage healthy tissue. It puts the body on an aging fast-track and you need to nip it in the bud. Symptoms may include:

★ Ongoing joint or muscle pain
★ Allergies, food intolerances, asthma
★ Gut disorders
★ Skin problems: lines, acne, eczema, dry eyes
★ Constant fatigue, exhaustion

GO CYY: Deinflame your body. Up your omega-3s (oily fish, flaxseed, chia seeds, nuts), add turmeric and ginger to food or juice, avoid foods to which you may be intolerant (gluten, soy, dairy, sugar, processed foods, alcohol). Eat alkaline (green veg) and organic if you can, including sprouted food and green juices. Reduce stress: Breathe, relax! (See page 30 for an inflammation case study.)

RECIPES TO TRY: Jolly green giant alkalizer, Scrambled eggs with turmeric, Zucchini spaghetti with squid; (see pages 42, 38, and 114).

wheatgrass, spinach, kale, sea vegetables, ginger, and perhaps add cayenne pepper (whatever you have around). Chewing on natural licorice sticks a couple of times a week is good, too. Drink calming teas: camomile, lemon balm. Do your CYY Breathing (see page 18). And then work out what your stress is and do everything possible to minimize its effects.

RECIPES TO TRY: Mixed seed crackers; Salmon and salsa "sandwiches" with quinoa (see pages 53 and 112).

FEET

★ If you notice very rough, dry skin on the heels you may need to support your thyroid (which is pretty much always a good idea anyway).

GO CYY: Eat seaweed, seafood, and vegetables for iodine, and selenium-rich sunflower seeds, eggs, and grains.

RECIPES TO TRY: Popcorn with seaweed salad, my sushi rolls (see pages 96 and 87 to 90).

GLUTEN INTOLERANCE

★ If small blisters appear on your arms, legs, or buttocks, it could be a sign of gluten-intolerance.

GO CYY: Stop eating gluten—in wheat, barley, buckwheat, rye, spelt, and commercially baked goods and cereals—for a couple of weeks. If the blisters go, you may need to readjust your diet long term.

RECIPES TO TRY: Crustless roast vegetable tart; Blueberry chia pancakes; Avocado and spicy tofu nori rolls (see pages 98, 34, and 87).

GUT PROBLEMS

★ Do you suffer from *general digestive problems* (bloating, diarrhea, constipation, gas), fatigue, allergies, athlete's foot, dandruff, skin problems (including eczema), mood swings, irritability, sugar cravings, or low immunity? Then you may have *candida*, a chronic yeast infection due to overgrowth of *Candida albicans* in the gut.

GO CYY: Avoid sugar (honey, syrups, most fruits, alcohol), and dairy (to cut out lactose), processed food, preservatives, and additives, all of which contain sugar. Avoid yeast and mushrooms (except those listed). Avoid rice cakes! Eat veg; fish; whole grains; legumes; garlic; shiitake and maitake

HOW DO YOU KNOW IF YOUR ADRENALS ARE STRESSED? SHINE A LIGHT IN YOUR EYE AND, IF IT STAYS DILATED, YOU HAVE AN ADRENAL PROBLEM ...

mushrooms. Try probiotics to restore good bacteria, and oregano, caprylic acid, and grapefruit seed extract to kill candida. (See page 28 for a candida case study.)

RECIPES TO TRY: Red lentil and cashew soup; Cod Provençal; Cauliflower and vegetable paella (see pages 61, 118, and 113).

★ If you feel you aren't digesting food properly, are burping, or feel heavy or tight after a meal, it may be because you have low stomach acidity. *Test*: Take a spoon of cider vinegar in water before a meal. If your stomach burns, that's good. If not, your stomach acidity may need a boost, so take the vinegar solution before every meal for a while.

GO CYY: Make sure you chew food properly to start the digestive process. Eat therapeutic, digestion-friendly spices (fennel, cardamom, pepper, horseradish, ginger), and foods high in digestive enzymes, such as pineapple and papaya.

RECIPES TO TRY: Moroccan spicy lentil stew; Quinoa maki rolls; Carrot, pear, and ginger slice (see pages 97, 89, and 149).

★ *fine lines above the eyebrows* can signify gut stress. A detox can clean your intestines.

GO CYY: Try a four-day cleanse: Take out anything inflammatory (dairy, wheat, sugar, meat, alcohol, caffeine) and eat nutrient-dense, high-fiber veggies instead. Add probiotic foods (miso, sauerkraut) and drink lots of water. Take psyllium husks to help cleanse and add a L-glutamine supplement to heal the gut and increase youthfulness.

RECIPES TO TRY: Gardener's pie; Tomato jellies; Butternut and carrot soup (see pages 104, 84, and 55).

★ *slow transit time in the gut* can be an issue; in other words, if you are not passing a stool at least once a day, you could find yourself with anything from bowel pockets to diverticulitis to IBS.

GO CYY: Figure out if you are dehydrated, if you eat too little fiber, or too many processed foods. Good recipes to choose from are anything containing chia seeds.

RECIPES TO TRY: Quinoa oatmeal with pear and cinnamon; Mixed seed crackers; Quick berry jam with chia seeds (see pages 37, 53, and 33).

HAIR

★ If it's dry, splitting, graying, receding, falling out, or you have dandruff, you may need to increase vitamin B-12 and iron. Or it may be that your gut is not absorbing nutrients properly (see page 20). Also look at stress levels and thyroid function if you have thinning hair.

GO CYY: For vitamin B-12: eat liver, sardines, trout, salmon. Vegetarians can try eggs and nutritional yeast (buy B-12 fortified varieties). For iron: Eat edamame beans, dark green leafy veg (kale, watercress, spinach), lentils, quinoa, kidney, pinto, and black-eye peas, potatoes, eggs, beet, sesame seeds, dried fruit.

RECIPES TO TRY: Salmon and salsa "sandwiches" with quinoa; Beet, sweet potato, and quinoa burger (see pages 112 and 108).

ARE YOU ACIDIC?

If you eat too many acid-producing foods you may experience:

★ Dry, wrinkled skin; dull (sometimes falling out) hair; thin nails that split easily

★ Joint stiffness, osteoarthritis, gout (due to a build up of uric acid)

★ Tiredness, low mood, mental slowness, lack of energy

★ Digestive disorders

★ Weakened bones, osteoporosis

GO CYY: To alkalize your body so you start to feel young again, eat 80 percent alkaline food to 20 percent acid-forming foods. That means wolfing down green veg, sprouted foods, nut milks, seeds, legumes (chickpeas, lentils), beans, avocado, and olive oil. Avoid red meat, dairy, caffeine, sugar, preservatives, and alcohol. See page 16 for more. (And see page 29 for an acidity case study.)

RECIPES TO TRY: Nutty white soup; Steamed Asian fragrant fish with sesame broccoli (see pages 60 and 118).

INSOMNIA

★ Sleep deprivation is seriously aging. It affects metabolism and energy levels. You feel hungrier and eat more sugary and fatty foods but are also less tolerant to them, thus increasing the risk of obesity and diabetes. Cortisol levels are higher, accelerating the aging process. Memory is impaired, healing less efficient, the immune system falters. Skin starts to look older, lined, and less taut.

Some foods contribute to insomnia: caffeine, soft drinks, alcohol, or a diet high in sugar and refined carbs, which triggers the "fight or flight" response, keeping you on alert.

GO CYY: Don't eat too late; by 7.30 p.m. on normal days. Avoid natural stimulants (see above). Eat foods high in tryptophan, a sleep-inducing amino acid. Try spirulina, spinach, oily fish, eggs, pumpkin seeds, almonds, bananas, chicken, and turkey. Keep stress low (exercise and do CYY Breathing, to reduce adrenal overload). Aim for eight hours sleep and go to bed before 11 p.m. so your body can detox when it should. If you can't, catch up through naps.

RECIPE TO TRY: Indian fish curry (see page 116).

JOINT PAIN

★ this may be caused by *overacidity* creating an *inflammatory* response. So alkalize, alkalize, alkalize (see page 16).

GO CYY: Juice and eat green leafy veg, eat legumes and nonacid forming grains (amaranth, buckwheat, millet, or quinoa). Take anti-inflammatory turmeric (in juices or stews). Avoid acid-forming meat, dairy, sugar, and alcohol.

RECIPES TO TRY: Cauliflower and vegetable paella, Split pea dhal, Moroccan spicy lentil stew (see pages 103, 113, and 97).

LIPS

★ If *dry* or *cracked*, your *gut* may be *irritated* or *inflamed*. Cracks at the side of the mouth may indicate a vitamin B-12 deficiency.

GO CYY: For vitamin B-12: eat liver and oily fish. Veggies can try eggs and nutritional yeast (B-12 fortified). To soothe the gut: eat veg and fruit (bran or high-fiber cereals can be harsh on an inflamed gut). Eat ginger and turmeric and drink ginger and peppermint teas.

RECIPES TO TRY: Salmon and salsa "sandwiches" with quinoa; French onion soup (see pages 112 and 58).

LOW IMMUNITY

★ If it takes 10 days for a cut to heal, if you get low-grade infections (colds, sniffles, cold sores) all the time, or if you've recently taken a course of antibiotics—which can kill off the protective, friendly bacteria in your gut—then your immune system definitely needs a boost. Good immunity is crucial for good youthing: There are 100 trillion bacteria living in and on your body and keeping them in the right balance is what makes your immune system robust.

GO CYY: 70% of the immune system is in the lining of the intestines, so get gut flora in shape by eating fermented foods and plain yogurt which contain rebalancing *Bifidobacteria* and *Lactobacillus* probiotics. Up your intake of garlic, enriching greens (chlorella, spirulina), oily fish and seafood, pumpkin seeds, eggs, mushrooms, and Brazils (all high in selenium and zinc). Look to your vitamins too: Foods high in vitamins B, C, and D (green veg and citrus) will help. During and after a course of antibiotics, always take probiotic supplements to restore gut and immune health.

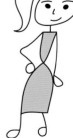

Rice cakes may be low in calories but they process as if they were a chocolate bar, putting fat on your liver and disturbing your blood sugar balance.

RECIPES TO TRY: Gardener's Pie, Aromatic mackerel and fennel salad, Chia tabbouleh (see pages 104, 63, and 76).

LOW MOOD

★ If you're *feeling low*, you may notice extreme *fatigue, poor appetite, insomnia,* and inability to concentrate. Nutrient deficiency can lead to depression and a nutrient-dense, fiber-rich diet can help sort it out; after all, 90 percent of the body's serotonin is produced in the digestive tract.

GO CYY: Avoid alcohol. Check for food allergies (see page 22). Up your B vitamins (especially B-12 and folic acid), and omega-3 fatty acids by eating nuts and seeds (especially Brazils and hemp seeds), nutritional yeast (B-12 fortified), beans, lentils, asparagus, oily fish, chlorella, and spirulina. And don't forget to exercise for those "happy hormones."

RECIPES TO TRY: Waldorf salad with mayonnaise; Juice twice daily; Almond butter (see pages 66, 41 to 46, and 82).

NAILS

★ If ridged or pale, it may show iron or calcium deficiency.

GO CYY: For calcium: eat seaweed, kale, and deep green veg, parsley, watercress, almonds, Brazil nuts, and pecans. For iron, see "Hair" (page 24).

RECIPES TO TRY: Beet salsa; Avocado, cauliflower, and spicy tofu nori rolls (see pages 126 and 87).

★ If you have white spots on your nails, you might like to look at boosting your levels of zinc.

GO CYY: Eat pumpkin and sesame seeds, pecans, Brazils, and walnuts, salmon, gingerroot, whole grains, rye, oats.

RECIPES TO TRY: Special guacamole; Pecan pies (see pages 126 and 143).

PMS (PREMENSTRUAL SYNDROME)

★ Distressing, but quite common. You may get spots, breast tenderness, bloating, swollen hands and feet, irritability, pelvic and back pain, mood swings, and low energy. In the vast majority of cases, eating CYY will diminish symptoms and leave you feeling energetic all month. A very youthing way to be.

✳ ✳ ✳

BRUSH YOUR SKIN
I can't say it often enough: daily skin brushing is one of the best youthing tools. It rejuvenates you inside and out. It leaves skin soft and smooth (you'll notice a difference within a week). It stimulates the lymph (good for immunity and detox) and increases the blood supply to the gut (good for improved digestion and nutrient transfer).

HOW TO DO IT: Use a soft bristle brush. Starting on the soles of the feet, briskly brush skin in a clockwise circular motion toward the heart. Cover the whole body (except the face). This will take two to three minutes a day: do it before a shower or bath. Lather yourself with shea butter to finish and make your skin super smooth.

✳ ✳ ✳

GO CYY: Stop eating salt and animal fats (dairy and meat) and eat fiber- and B vitamin-rich leafy greens, beans, lentils, nuts, whole grains, and root veg. For hot flushes, avoid "heating" meat, salt, sugar, alcohol, garlic, or onion.

RECIPES TO TRY: "Cheesy" kale chips; Eggplant-coconut rolls (see pages 75 and 124).

SKIN

★ If wrinkled, dry, or with fine lines: you're probably not getting enough omega-3. Or you are dehydrated and lacking in silica and collagen (take these as supplements).

GO CYY: Eat more oily fish and seeds. Drink at least eight glasses of water a day (not including coffee and tea).

RECIPE TO TRY: Octopus salad (see page 69).

★ Red spots may signify too much meat, salt, or sugar.

GO CYY: Go veggie for a month; cut salt and refined sugar.

RECIPES TO TRY: Salad bouquet; Turmeric marinade; Chia tabbouleh (see pages 66, 83, and 76).

★ White spots may be dairy- or mucus-related.

GO CYY: If you eat cow's milk, try goat or sheep instead. Or cut out dairy for a few months and see if skin improves.

YOUR BEDROOM SHOULD BE A HAVEN OF REST, SO TAKE OUT THE TV AND ELECTRICAL GOODS, EVEN YOUR ALARM CLOCK

RECIPE TO TRY: Gardener's pie (see page 104).

★ If pale, you may have anemia due to lack of iron or B-12.

GO CYY: For foods rich in iron and vitamin B-12, try drinking ½ cup [125 ml] of wheatgrass juice daily and see "Hair" (page 24).

RECIPES TO TRY: Cauliflower maki rolls (see page 90). (Also see page 29 for a case study about improving skin.)

SWEATING

★ If you sweat a lot, you may need to strengthen the lungs, so they can help the skin. You might also need potassium, as it can be lost through sweat. The liver may be overheating, so avoid sugar, salt, red meat, and alcohol.

GO CYY: Eat cruciferous veg, onions, garlic, scallions, and potassium-rich avocado, beans, tomato, spinach, banana. Do CYY Breathing (see page 18) twice daily.

RECIPES TO TRY: Potato pancakes; Spelt pizza with scallions, artichokes, and rosemary (see pages 36 and 107).

VEINS

★ Broken "spider veins" in legs, chest, or face and "popping" veins in hands or legs can show a lack of flavonoids.

GO CYY: Eat buckwheat, apples, asparagus, figs, and citrus to raise flavonoid levels and strengthen venous integrity.

NB: If you suspect varicose veins (deep raised veins which can be seen through the skin), consult your doctor.

RECIPE TO TRY: Fig slice (see page 149).

* * *

DESTRESS IS BEST
★ Join a yoga or pilates class
★ Do CYY Breathing (see page 18)
★ Refuse to work during weekends and evenings
★ Get eight hours' sleep (starting at least one hour before midnight)
★ Try hard not to be anxious (meditation and mindfulness can help)
★ Laugh a lot

* * *

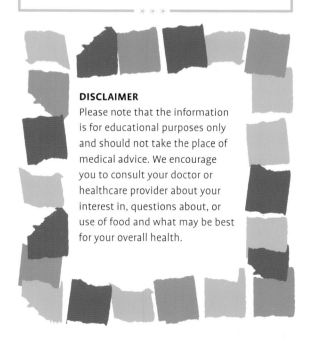

DISCLAIMER
Please note that the information is for educational purposes only and should not take the place of medical advice. We encourage you to consult your doctor or healthcare provider about your interest in, questions about, or use of food and what may be best for your overall health.

> ‘My soul is dark with stormy riot,
> Directly traceable to diet.’
>
> SAMUEL HOFFENSTEIN, SCREENWRITER

INFLAMMATION

Jacquetta was 62 when she came to see me with severe arthritic pain in her feet. She was of Italian heritage, small and round, but with no signs of diabetes or high blood pressure. She had swollen feet—for which she'd been given diuretics by her doctor—along with high inflammatory markers in her blood which showed "something was going on," as the doctor put it.

She was in pain most of the time and so had started comfort eating: processed foods, cakes, and cookies. Being Italian, she also cooked tomatoes, eggplants, and peppers almost every day. She'd fry these in processed cooking oils. Worried about water retention and swollen feet, she barely drank any liquids. As a result her kidneys were not able to filter or flush properly and acids and toxins were being deposited in her joints, hands, and feet, causing increasing inflammation, and—it soon became clear—gout (where uric acid crystals accumulate in joints).

We needed to break the cycle. With chronic inflammation, the immune system is on constant alert. This means there are high levels of the stress hormone cortisol (see right). It is linked to accelerated aging (in skin, nails, hair, muscles, bones, memory, and lowered energy) and to increased fat deposits around the middle.

Jacquetta tried an anti-inflammatory diet for a month (see below). Within a week she lost seven pounds, but her joint pain was more intense. After three weeks, the pain started to lessen. It took six months before she was pain-free. I worried she might go back to comfort eating, but by then she had lost 6.3 kg [14 lb] and had noticed increased energy; stronger joints; tauter skin; and better immunity.

Fighting inflammation is hugely important for youthing, because it doesn't just happen in the joints. It can dispose the brain to develop Alzheimer's disease.

---

* * *

**TOO MUCH CORTISOL?
SIGNS AND SYMPTOMS**
★ Dry, dull skin, hair, and nails
★ Weight gain around the waist
★ Food cravings and/ or allergies
★ Lack of energy
★ Muscle weakness
★ High blood pressure
★ Difficulty sleeping
★ Tension and irritability
★ Difficulty concentrating, poor memory

* * *

---

* * *

JACQUETTA'S ANTI-INFLAMMATORY DIET
★ Cut out eggplants, peppers, potatoes, tomatoes; common allergens such as wheat, dairy, soy, or shellfish; refined sugars
★ Cook only with coconut or avocado oils
★ If you have gout, avoid bacon, liver, kidneys, and alcohol
★ Eat a wide range of veg, fruits (especially berries), seaweeds, beans
★ Eat MSM-rich alfalfa sprouts, radishes, apples, bananas, strawberries
★ Get omega-3 fatty acids from oily fish, nuts, and seeds
★ Add anti-inflammatory turmeric, ginger, and garlic to dishes
★ Drink eight glasses of water a day

* * *

Inflammation is your body's first call for action. It is saying "I am overburdened and in contact with something that is dangerous, please remove it or I will continue to inflame." It is trying to get you to pay attention.

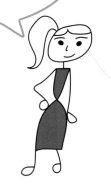

YOUR BEDROOM SHOULD BE A HAVEN OF REST, SO TAKE OUT THE TV AND ELECTRICAL GOODS, EVEN YOUR ALARM CLOCK

RECIPE TO TRY: Gardener's pie (see page 104).

★ If pale, you may have anemia due to lack of iron or B-12.

GO CYY: For foods rich in iron and vitamin B-12, try drinking ½ cup [125 ml] of wheatgrass juice daily and see "Hair" (page 24).

RECIPES TO TRY: Cauliflower maki rolls (see page 90). (Also see page 29 for a case study about improving skin.)

SWEATING

★ If you sweat a lot, you may need to strengthen the lungs, so they can help the skin. You might also need potassium, as it can be lost through sweat. The liver may be overheating, so avoid sugar, salt, red meat, and alcohol.

GO CYY: Eat cruciferous veg, onions, garlic, scallions, and potassium-rich avocado, beans, tomato, spinach, banana. Do CYY Breathing (see page 18) twice daily.

RECIPES TO TRY: Potato pancakes; Spelt pizza with scallions, artichokes, and rosemary (see pages 36 and 107).

VEINS

★ Broken "spider veins" in legs, chest, or face and "popping" veins in hands or legs can show a lack of flavonoids.

GO CYY: Eat buckwheat, apples, asparagus, figs, and citrus to raise flavonoid levels and strengthen venous integrity.

NB: If you suspect varicose veins (deep raised veins which can be seen through the skin), consult your doctor.

RECIPE TO TRY: Fig slice (see page 149).

* * *

DESTRESS IS BEST
★ Join a yoga or pilates class
★ Do CYY Breathing (see page 18)
★ Refuse to work during weekends and evenings
★ Get eight hours' sleep (starting at least one hour before midnight)
★ Try hard not to be anxious (meditation and mindfulness can help)
★ Laugh a lot

* * *

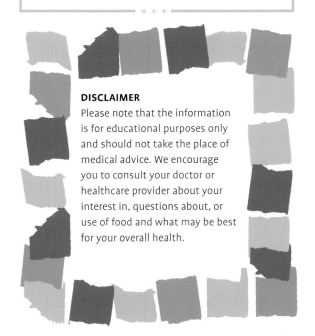

DISCLAIMER
Please note that the information is for educational purposes only and should not take the place of medical advice. We encourage you to consult your doctor or healthcare provider about your interest in, questions about, or use of food and what may be best for your overall health.

I Want to Start a Youthing Revolution

Every day, I meet people whose lives (and bodies) are transformed when they make youthing changes to what they cook. (All names have been changed.) I hope these case studies inspire you to change your life and body, too. If so, tell the person next to you. Then the revolution will begin.

DIGESTION

Good digestion is key to youthing. Working well, it provides an age-defying phytonutrient, vitamin, and mineral feast that revitalizes your system. When it underperforms, you're on an antiyouthing roller coaster and chronic fatigue, undernourished muscles, skin, hair, and nails, headaches, a shaky immune system, weight issues, depression, high cholesterol, and diabetes can result.

Coleen was 32, she had severe bloating and painful spasms within 30 minutes of eating and alternated between constipation and diarrhea. Her skin was blotchy. She had colds every few weeks and felt run down. Her mood was low, sometimes volatile. She thought the symptoms had come on since she'd vacationed in Thailand a year ago. She'd had food poisoning there and, on her return, contracted a throat infection that required two courses of antibiotics.

It seemed clear that Coleen had candidiasis. It's common after taking antibiotics because they destroy both "good" and "bad" bacteria, unbalancing the gut's ecosystem and allowing candida to grow unchecked. She did a stool test and this was the case. The infection had traveled from intestines to anus, where it was causing itching. Coleen had also developed dandruff, which was connected.

We attacked in two stages. The first was to lighten the load on the gut with a 24-hour veg juice detox. After that, Coleen stuck to the anticandida diet for one month, taking slippery elm, charcoal, and psyllium husks to soothe the digestive tract; antifungal caprylic acid and oregano, milk thistle, and dandelion for liver support, and a strong full-spectrum probiotic. The anticandida diet cuts refined and other sugars and boosts gut bacteria with nutrient-dense, high-fiber foods, killing off the fungal jungle with herbs. Coleen struggled with it at first, but when I gave her tasty recipes, her whole family started eating more healthily.

After a month she looked and felt revitalized. The bloating and spasms disappeared. She felt brighter, plus her sleep and energy levels had improved. She'd lost weight and people told her she looked younger, healthier, and happier.

I'd advise sticking to this diet for six months and taking probiotics daily. Coleen didn't see this as a hardship: Her family were enjoying this healthy, youthing way of eating and were all feeling more upbeat. That's youthing 1, candida 0.

---

* * *

CANDIDA: SIGNS AND SYMPTOMS

★ Bloating, digestive complaints, discomfort after eating
★ Thrush, dandruff
★ Craving for sugar and starch
★ Low immune system, frequent low-grade illnesses
★ Headaches, mild depression
★ Overweight

* * *

---

* * *

COLEEN'S ANTICANDIDA DIET

★ Cut out coffee, tea, dairy, wheat, preservatives, additives, yeast, mushrooms, sugar (plus fruit and juice), and alcohol
★ Start the day with hot water and lemon
★ Eat vegetables and juice them
★ Include sprouted vegetables (broccoli, chive, cress, mustard, onion, radish) and beans
★ Eat protein (though eat mostly plants with a little fish)
★ Eat antifungal garlic, cinnamon, fennel, lemon grass, licorice
★ Drink water and herbal tea
★ Try my recipes; most are anticandida, but avoid any with fruit, yeast, or maple syrup

* * *

> ‘Happiness: a good bank account,
> a good cook, and a good digestion,’
>
> JEAN-JACQUES ROUSSEAU

ALKALIZE

To keep brain and body young, I always advise people to alkalize. To recap, this is a way of helping your body balance to a slightly alkaline pH, so everything works at its youthing optimum. Eating acid-forming foods (the worst culprits are meat, dairy, coffee, cola, refined, and processed foods) makes this harder, making the body susceptible to aging. If that's not enough, overacidity also keeps you fat!

Stephen came to see me saying he was only there because his wife insisted. He said he was tired, but slept well; he had put on weight though he was eating the same food. He was beginning to feel his age (40!), but otherwise there was nothing much wrong. Could I "fix" him? He was overweight and looked puffy. He had rings under his eyes, dull hair, and pale, clammy skin. His eyes were bright and anxious. He was buzzing internally, yet his body was still.

It was clear he was suffering. He didn't want to diet, in fact was resistant to making changes. So I told him what he wanted to hear: that he was in pretty good shape. However, he could speed his weight loss by taking dairy out of his diet (dairy is acid-forming and he'd told me this was a food he ate too much). And so he stopped. He didn't want to juice, so took an algae and chlorella mix in the mornings (from health food stores). Within two weeks he had lost weight and most of the aging "puffiness" and came back for more youthing advice.

We discussed options and eventually he agreed to come off wheat and start eating 40 percent raw food to boost his alkalinity. After a couple of weeks his energy levels soared, his cheeks gained color, his skin was glowing, his hair was shinier. He felt happy, he said, for the first time in years. He looked 10 years younger (and a lot less grumpy). This, I thought, is youthing alkalization at work.

REINVENT YOUR SKIN

People always say how much better their skin looks after alkalizing for a couple of months. It's not just that pimples, acne, blotchiness, and skin irritations disappear (though they do). It's that the quality of the skin—texture, strength, and softness to the touch—is vastly improved.

This is for two reasons. First, the body rids itself of acids through skin, so skin conditions caused by overacidity (spots to rosacea to eczema) melt away. Secondly, an alkalizing diet is low in the simple sugars that cause collagen fibers to break. As collagen strengthens, skin gets more resilient.

* * *

A GOOD WAY TO ALKALIZE

STEP 1: For two weeks, stop eating dairy and meat, and start a daily green juice or take blue-green algae/chlorella with water and lemon juice.

STEP 2: For two months, eat 80 percent alkaline/20 percent acidic foods and also make 40 percent of your food intake raw (see page 16). Avoid wheat, cook only with avocado or coconut oils, and eat eggs, fish, or tofu a couple of times a week.

STEP 3: To maintain for life, eat 70 percent alkaline/30 percent acidic foods; easy if you eat 40 percent raw (see page 16).

* * *

Skeptics make the best patients, because once they see results they "get it" so completely and spread the word like no one else.

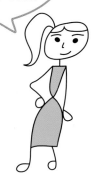

> 'My soul is dark with stormy riot,
> Directly traceable to diet.'
>
> SAMUEL HOFFENSTEIN, SCREENWRITER

INFLAMMATION

Jacquetta was 62 when she came to see me with severe arthritic pain in her feet. She was of Italian heritage, small and round, but with no signs of diabetes or high blood pressure. She had swollen feet—for which she'd been given diuretics by her doctor—along with high inflammatory markers in her blood which showed "something was going on," as the doctor put it.

She was in pain most of the time and so had started comfort eating: processed foods, cakes, and cookies. Being Italian, she also cooked tomatoes, eggplants, and peppers almost every day. She'd fry these in processed cooking oils. Worried about water retention and swollen feet, she barely drank any liquids. As a result her kidneys were not able to filter or flush properly and acids and toxins were being deposited in her joints, hands, and feet, causing increasing inflammation, and—it soon became clear—gout (where uric acid crystals accumulate in joints).

We needed to break the cycle. With chronic inflammation, the immune system is on constant alert. This means there are high levels of the stress hormone cortisol (see right). It is linked to accelerated aging (in skin, nails, hair, muscles, bones, memory, and lowered energy) and to increased fat deposits around the middle.

Jacquetta tried an anti-inflammatory diet for a month (see below). Within a week she lost seven pounds, but her joint pain was more intense. After three weeks, the pain started to lessen. It took six months before she was pain-free. I worried she might go back to comfort eating, but by then she had lost 6.3 kg [14 lb] and had noticed increased energy; stronger joints; tauter skin; and better immunity.

Fighting inflammation is hugely important for youthing, because it doesn't just happen in the joints. It can dispose the brain to develop Alzheimer's disease.

---

* * *

TOO MUCH CORTISOL?
SIGNS AND SYMPTOMS

★ Dry, dull skin, hair, and nails
★ Weight gain around the waist
★ Food cravings and/or allergies
★ Lack of energy
★ Muscle weakness
★ High blood pressure
★ Difficulty sleeping
★ Tension and irritability
★ Difficulty concentrating, poor memory

* * *

---

* * *

JACQUETTA'S ANTI-INFLAMMATORY DIET

★ Cut out eggplants, peppers, potatoes, tomatoes; common allergens such as wheat, dairy, soy, or shellfish; refined sugars
★ Cook only with coconut or avocado oils
★ If you have gout, avoid bacon, liver, kidneys, and alcohol
★ Eat a wide range of veg, fruits (especially berries), seaweeds, beans
★ Eat MSM-rich alfalfa sprouts, radishes, apples, bananas, strawberries
★ Get omega-3 fatty acids from oily fish, nuts, and seeds
★ Add anti-inflammatory turmeric, ginger, and garlic to dishes
★ Drink eight glasses of water a day

* * *

Inflammation is your body's first call for action. It is saying "I am overburdened and in contact with something that is dangerous, please remove it or I will continue to inflame." It is trying to get you to pay attention.

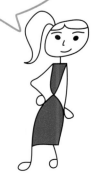

> 'Life expectancy would grow by leaps and bounds if green vegetables smelled as good as bacon,'
>
> DOUG LARSON, NEWSPAPER COLUMNIS

FOOD CONFUSION

Ellie, 26, came to talk about her skin (spots, eczema) and how fat and anxious she felt compared to her friends, who were supertoned and gorgeous (she said). It didn't seem fair as she went to the gym three times a week, slept nine to 10 hours a night, and ate only super-good-for-her foods. I was intrigued and asked for a rundown of them: Breakfast: Smoothie of chocolate whey protein powder, with added green algae powder occasionally. Snacks: Rice cakes, salami or carpaccio; daily energy or raw food bar (always after a workout); more whey protein in soy milk for an energy boost. Lunch and dinner: She's not often hungry but eats high-protein, low-carb, low-cal foods: chicken with veg, steak with salad, sushi with rice. With the odd dessert. Going out: Two glasses of white wine most nights. On big nights (twice a week), at least four vodkas with juice.

You can see why Ellie thinks she is healthy. But almost everything she eats has been mucked around with, bunged full of additives, put into packages, and sold back to her as a healthy miracle. Except it's not. Rice cakes, processed meats, energy bars, reconstituted whey powder, and processed soy milk are in truth junk foods, best avoided. Even sushi rice is packed full of sugar.

It's no wonder Ellie can't lose weight: she is a sugar monster. I checked one of her energy and raw bars: sugars made up 37 percent. Add to that her alcohol intake, which turns to sugar in the body. The foods were instrumental in creating not just her health problems, but also her anxiety. A high-sugar diet is an aging time bomb. It is antiyouthing for skin. It whacks your hormones—which is why Ellie has spots and sleeps for too long—causes mood fluctuations and, of course, blood sugar swings. I told Ellie to junk this "healthy" regime and eat foods as close as possible to their natural state; that's brown rice, not rice cakes.

We came up with a youth-proofing plan that would set her up for a long and healthy life and make her feel awesome now. She cut the pseudohealthy bars and powders (and anything else with more than 10 ingredients), and started eating plant-based, nutrient-rich, and fad-free, but still high-protein and low-carb. She loved to snack, so I gave her some recipes (see pages 71 to 76).

The amazing thing was that Ellie was able to stick to this new regime. The last time Ellie came to see me it was to say goodbye. She was happy: She'd stopped obsessing about her body and didn't feel the need to compare herself unfavorably to anyone. She was a good 10 pounds leaner, with glowing, blemish-free skin, a mane of glossy hair, and a new inner confidence that will set her up for life. My thought? You're never too young to start youthing ...

* * *

ELLIE'S NEW TAKE ON HEALTHY

★ Breakfast: Grind hemp seeds and use in veg smoothies; make your own protein-rich nut milks; eat beans and legumes

★ Lunch: Cook high-protein whole grains (such as quinoa) at the start of the week and dress up with different salad/veg. Take a can of tuna, houmous, or boiled eggs and Mixed seed crackers (see page 53) to the office

★ Dinner: When eating out, have fish or veg in Thai and Indian; anything (except tempura) in Japanese; the roast veg / beany option in Italian. Anywhere else, double up on protein "sides" and whack in some greens, too

* * *

If you do hard workouts and don't want to lose muscle as you age, eat 3¼ oz [90 g] protein a day instead of the recommended 1½ oz [45 g], preferably from plant-based sources.

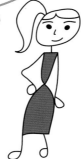

1

BREAKFASTS

'All happiness depends on a
leisurely breakfast,
JOHN GUNTHER

Fruit salad with ginger juice and orange

Mixing seeds (protein and fat) with fruit means this is a balanced protein and carbohydrate meal, the best start to the day. Don't worry too much about the types of fruit; try grapes, apricots, peaches, nectarines, mandarins, or passion fruits. Add coconut or almond milk or cream, if you want, or a topping of ground almonds and oats mixed with yogurt. **SERVES 6**

1¼ Tbsp sunflower seeds

1 apple, cored and chopped

1 pear, cored and sliced

1 orange, peeled and segmented, segments halved, plus juice of 1 orange

3 kiwis, peeled and quartered

1 papaya, peeled and chopped

1 mango, peeled and chopped

1¼ Tbsp pumpkin seeds

1¼ oz [37 g] nuts (whichever you like), chopped

1 thumb of gingerroot

1 If you want to roast the sunflower seeds, preheat the oven to 350°F [180°C], spread the seeds on a baking sheet, and bake for about 20 minutes so they roast and the oils are released. Watch carefully, so they don't catch and burn.

2 Mix the prepared fruits together, adding the seeds and nuts, then juice the ginger and add it to the fruit with the orange juice.

3 Cover and store in the refrigerator; it will last for five or six days.

Quick berry jam with chia seeds

Chia seeds are high in omega-3 fatty acids and minerals, great for the gut and at reducing cholesterol and blood pressure. Spread this on Mixed seed crackers (see page 53) for a seriously tasty and see-you-through-to-lunch breakfast. **MAKES 1 LARGE BOWL**

¾ cup [100 g] fresh or frozen blackberries

scant 1 cup [100 g] fresh or frozen raspberries

⅓ cup [50 g] fresh or frozen blueberries

½ tsp vanilla powder or seeds of ½ vanilla bean

a few dates, pitted, finely chopped, to taste (optional)

¼ cup chia seeds

1 Put the berries in a pan and just cover with about 7 Tbsp [100 ml] of filtered water. Heat gently and add the vanilla. Let it bubble gently until it starts to turn into a sauce.

2 Taste and add the dates, to sweeten, if using. Take off the heat and stir in the chia seeds. Chill for a few hours and eat within five days.

3 To make a version of this even more quickly, just blend fresh berries with chia and vanilla to make a raw jam. The color will fade, so eat it immediately.

Oat pancakes with apple and cashews

A weekend treat. Maple syrup is high in sugar but also in minerals such as manganese, which is great for bones and skin.
MAKES 8

1 Blitz the oats in a blender. Pour them into a bowl with the baking powder. Make a well in the center and drop in the oil, egg, and milk. Whisk, drawing in the dry ingredients to make a smooth batter.

2 Heat two frying pans over medium-low heat and wipe with coconut oil. Lay the apple and cashews in one pan. Drop 1 Tbsp of the batter into the other (you might be able to cook three at a time, depending on pan size). Fry for one to two minutes, until bubbling. Flip and fry for another minute. Stir the apple and cashews, then pour in the syrup. Heat for 30 seconds, then remove and keep warm while you cook all the pancakes. Serve with the apple and cashews.

1½ cups [125 g] jumbo oats

1½ tsp gluten-free baking powder

1 Tbsp coconut oil, melted, plus more to cook

1 large egg, lightly beaten

½ cup [125 ml] almond milk

1 apple, cored and sliced

2 Tbsp cashews, chopped

1 Tbsp maple syrup (optional)

Blueberry chia pancakes

This antioxidant-rich pancake is a wake-up for all your cells. A great source of vitamin C and zinc, it's soothing for the gut, low in calories, high in nutrition, and will put a zing into your morning step. **MAKES 16**

1 The night before, sift the flour into a mixing bowl and whisk in the chia, baking powder, cinnamon, and salt. Make a well in the center and beat in the almond milk until you have a smooth batter. Beat in the vanilla and blueberries. Cover and chill overnight.

2 During the same evening, if you can, chill the coconut milk for a few hours. Remove the "cream" from the top and put it in a bowl. Add the cinnamon and syrup, then whip until smooth and creamy. Set aside.

3 Heat a large frying pan over medium heat and wipe with coconut oil. Drop in 1 Tbsp of the batter (you might be able to cook three at a time, depending on the size of your pan). When bubbles appear on the surface, flip over and cook for two minutes more, until golden and fluffy. Keep warm. Repeat to cook all the pancakes. Serve with the cinnamon cream.

FOR THE PANCAKES

scant 1 cup [100 g] spelt flour

2 Tbsp chia seeds

2 tsp baking powder

½ tsp ground cinnamon

pinch of Himalayan or Celtic salt

⅞ cup cup [200 ml] almond milk

1 tsp vanilla bean paste

⅓ cup [50 g] blueberries

2 tsp coconut oil

FOR THE CINNAMON CREAM

7 Tbsp [100 ml] coconut milk, ideally homemade (see page 46)

1 tsp ground cinnamon

1 Tbsp maple syrup (optional)

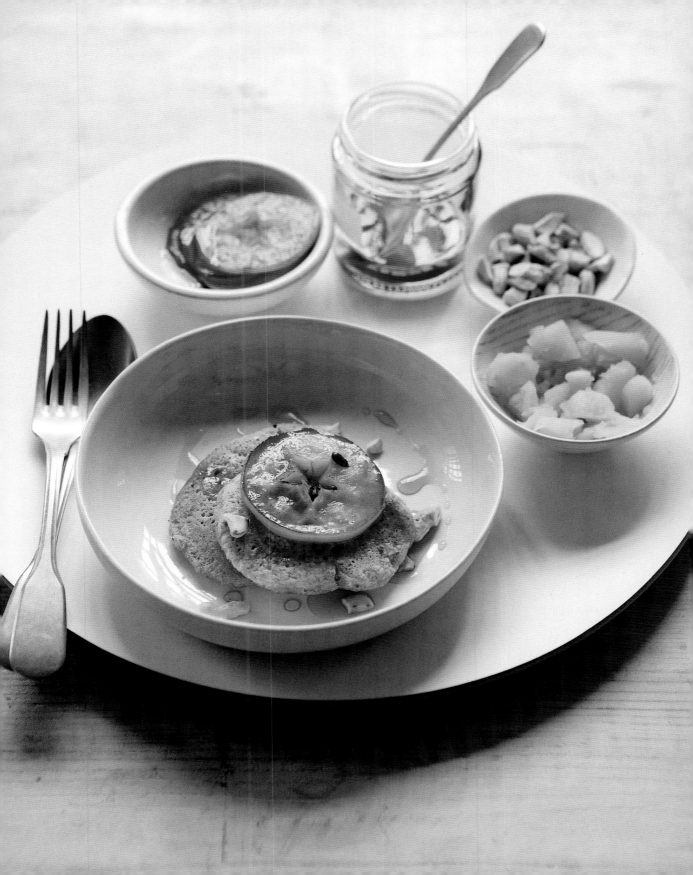

Potato pancakes

I love this savory gluten-free breakfast. It's dense enough to make you feel as if you've had a "fry-up," but light enough that you don't feel weighed down or sleepy afterward. Plus it's a good dairy-free mixture of carbohydrate and protein, so nicely youthing. **SERVES 4**

1 Boil and mash the potato. When cooled slightly, add the onion, flour, baking powder, and egg, then stir in the cashew milk and chives (if using). When combined well, let rest for about five minutes.

2 Heat the oil in a frying pan and, when it's hot, add 1 Tbsp of the potato mixture, slightly spreading to make it round. Add another one or two, depending on the size of your pan (the pancakes should not be crammed together). Fry for three to four minutes on either side, until golden brown. Set aside and keep warm while you cook the rest.

4¼ oz [125 g] mealy potato

½ onion, grated

scant ¼ cup [30 g] rice flour

½ tsp gluten-free baking powder

1 egg, lightly beaten

⅜ cup [90 ml] cashew milk, or other nut milk

1 Tbsp chopped chives (optional)

2 tsp coconut oil

Chia oatmeal with almond milk and berries

If you want to feel on top of your game while feeding your skin and cells, this is the breakfast for you. The vanilla is uplifting and the chia is hydrating and cleansing for the gut. Deliciously high in omegas and protein, this is an anti-inflammatory and alkalizing dream. **SERVES 1**

1 Soak the chia seeds in the almond milk for a minimum of two hours, or overnight in the refrigerator.

2 Stir in the vanilla until evenly mixed, then spoon into a serving bowl. Sprinkle over the almonds and berries to serve.

2 Tbsp chia seeds

generous 1 cup [250 ml] almond milk

½ tsp vanilla powder or extract, or seeds of ½ vanilla bean

1 Tbsp coarsely chopped almonds

handful of mixed berries

Quinoa oatmeal with vanilla and banana

Quinoa is a little gem: it dates back 4,000 years, contains all the essential amino acids, is high in fiber, rich in minerals, and raises energy levels. All of which makes this a great all-round youthing breakfast. **SERVES 1**

1 Put the ingredients into a pan with 5 Tbsp [75 ml] of filtered water. Cook gently until the water evaporates and the quinoa is hot through.

2 If you would like a creamier oatmeal, add a little hemp, cashew, or almond milk to serve.

⅓ cup [70 g] cooked quinoa (see page 89)

¼ tsp vanilla powder or ½ tsp vanilla extract, or seeds of ½ vanilla bean

1 Tbsp raisins

½ Tbsp coconut oil

½ banana, mashed

hemp, cashew, or almond milk, to serve (optional)

Quinoa oatmeal with pear and cinnamon

This is a perfect gluten-free, high-protein, and deliciously warming winter breakfast. It is also a fabulous way of using up any quinoa left over from the day before. **SERVES 1**

1 Add all the ingredients to a small pan and bring to a boil over medium to low heat. Reduce the heat and simmer gently for five to 10 minutes, until everything is well amalgamated and the consistency is to your liking.

2 Serve with a splash more cold almond milk, if you like.

⅓ cup [70 g] cooked quinoa (see page 89)

½ cup [125 ml] almond milk, plus more to serve (optional)

¼ tsp ground cinnamon

1 small pear, coarsely chopped

Scrambled egg breakfast muffins

A hugely youthing breakfast, this contains full amino acids (from eggs), immune-boosters (from shiitake mushrooms and onions), antioxidants (from spinach and tomatoes), and lots of lovely vitamins (including hard-to-get B12 in the nutritional yeast).
SERVES 4

6 dried shiitake mushrooms

1 tsp coconut oil

6 large eggs

3 scallions, thinly sliced

1¾ oz [50 g] baby spinach, shredded

2 Tbsp nutritional yeast flakes

2 tomatoes, flesh chopped,
seeds discarded

¼ tsp cayenne pepper

1 Put the shiitake in a small bowl and cover with just-boiled filtered water. Let soak for 30 minutes, then drain and finely chop.

2 Preheat the oven to 400°F [200°C]. Oil a six-section nonstick muffin pan with the coconut oil.

3 Whisk the eggs well and beat in the scallions, spinach, mushrooms, nutritional yeast, tomatoes, and cayenne. Divide between the muffin sections.

4 Bake for 20 to 25 minutes, until well risen. These are delicious hot or cold, so are a perfect packed lunch when you are on the go.

Scrambled eggs with turmeric

An anti-inflammatory, protein-rich breakfast. Lots of people love a morning egg and the ginger and turmeric add extra spice and goodness to help the body detox and digest. SERVES 1

1 Tbsp organic coconut milk, ideally homemade (see page 46), plus more if needed

½ tsp coconut oil

½ tsp ground turmeric

½ tsp minced gingerroot

3 eggs, lightly beaten

1 Spoon the coconut milk into a pan, add the coconut oil, turmeric, and ginger and place over medium heat. Let the milk simmer slowly until it becomes a thick base.

2 Add the eggs, with some more coconut milk if you wish. Cook the eggs to your preference.

3 Serve on sprouted bread toast for a substantial start to the day.

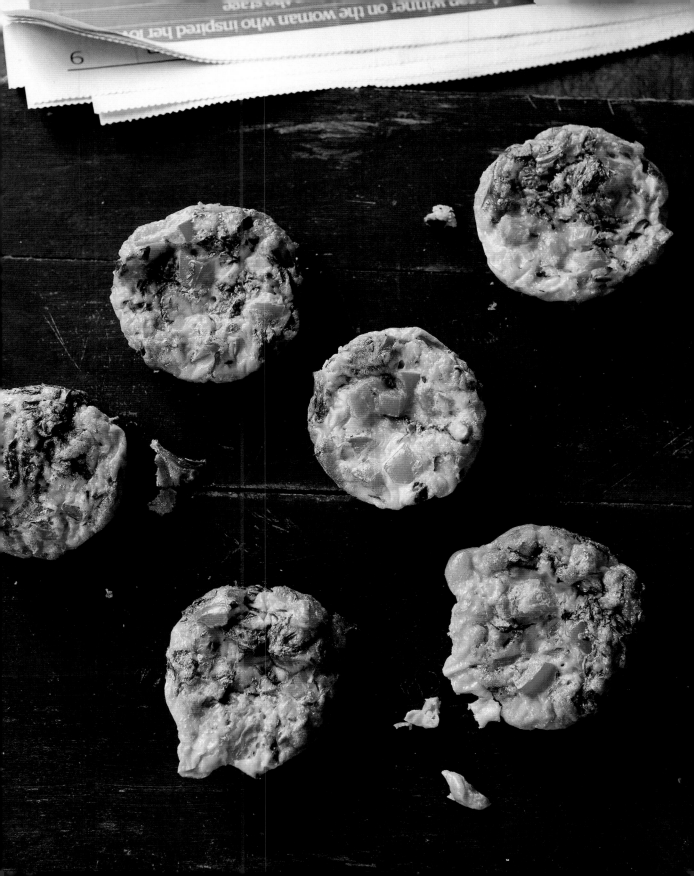

Baked "cheesy" eggs

A silky smooth, indulgent breakfast. Packed with protein and omega oils, this will raise your energy levels while giving you a lovely rich, "cheesy" comfort-food taste, even though it's entirely dairy-free. Delicious on its own, or with a Mixed seed cracker (see page 53). **SERVES 1**

1 Preheat the oven to 375°F [190°C].

2 Put the oil into a small pan, melt it, then throw in the spinach leaves and wilt for one minute only, to keep the spinach green. Stir in a pinch of nutmeg and some pepper. Put this into a ramekin. Now crack the egg straight in on top of the spinach.

3 Mix the yeast flakes with the cashew milk in a small bowl or cup, add more nutmeg and pepper to taste, and pour over the egg. Bake in the oven for 15 to 18 minutes. Check to see if the egg is still soft and the white around it is cooked by gently pressing. Put the ramekin onto a plate and sprinkle with chopped parsley. Serve immediately.

smidgen of coconut oil

handful of baby spinach

freshly grated nutmeg

freshly ground black pepper

1 large egg

pinch of nutritional yeast flakes

scant ¼ cup [50 ml] cashew milk, or other nut milk

2 Tbsp chopped parsley leaves

2

JUICES

'A fit, healthy body—that is the
best fashion statement,

JESS C SCOTT

Juices, smoothies, and shakes have become hugely popular, but I've noticed that most recipes contain a lot of natural sugars, usually in the form of fruit (fresh or dried) or sometimes added syrups. The recipes here are mostly veg, which means they're much healthier and won't give the body an antiyouthing sugar shock. Juices are highly nutritious. And don't throw away the veg waste; you can use it in stews and curries!

Making juices

Flow all the ingredients through the juicer, then drink at once (but slowly) to get the optimum nutritional and youthing benefits. These recipes here and overleaf all serve one, except where specified.

NOTE
The weight is of the vegetable or herb before it is juiced. Weigh veg (such as a zucchini) to find out if you need to use it all or just a fraction of it. If you're allergic to honey or bee stings, don't use bee pollen.

Vitamin burst

4 medium carrots

1 beet

4½ oz [130 g] cucumber

4 oz [115 g] cabbage

Jolly green giant alkalizer

leaves from 1 large Boston lettuce

juice of 1 lime

3½ oz [100 g] zucchini

⅓-oz [10-g] piece of gingerroot

3½ oz [100 g] spinach

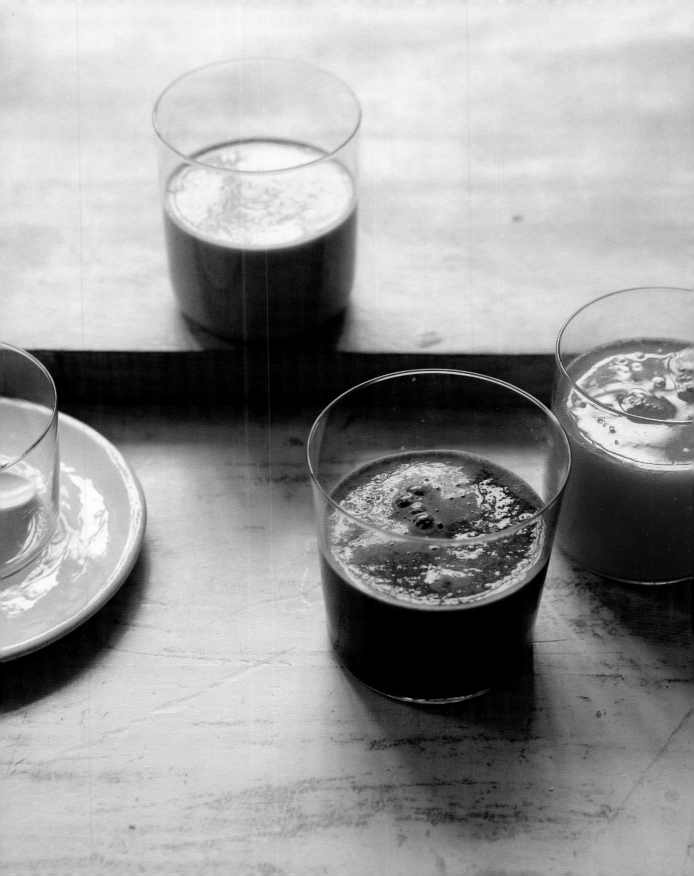

Detox juice

 V DF GF

7 oz [200 g] daikon

5¼ oz [150 g] fennel

1 oz [25 g] parsley

3 oz [80 g] spinach

juice of 1 lemon

1-oz [30-g] piece of gingerroot

Spicy vitamin A wake-up juice

 V DF GF

6 oz [170 g] daikon

11¼ oz [320 g] carrot

1-oz [30-g] piece of gingerroot

juice of 1 lime

Energy root green

 V DF GF

¼ cucumber

1 beet

2½ oz [70 g] spinach

1 apple

Breakfast shake

 V DF GF

MAKES 2 GLASSES

½ banana (1¾ oz/50 g)

scant ¼ cup [20 g] pumpkin seeds

scant ¼ cup [25 g] almonds

1 tsp bee pollen (optional)

generous 1 cup [250 ml] filtered water

Skin rejuvenator

 V DF GF

1¾ oz [50 g] sweet potato

8¾ oz [250 g] carrot

3½ oz [100 g] red bell pepper

juice of 1 lime

½ tsp ground turmeric

Hot winter warmer

The spicy, comforting tastes of midwinter are all here. Add a star anise or a clove for an extra mulled effect.

1 Juice the ginger and apple and pour ⅝ cup [150 ml] of boiling filtered water on top. Add ground cinnamon for an extra taste of cold weather comfort, if you want, which will also stabilize your blood sugar.

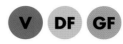

1-oz [30-g] piece of gingerroot

3½ oz [100 g] apple

a little ground cinnamon (optional)

Fast intense greens

You can buy spirulina and chlorella in powder form (add them to any of your juices for an extra bit of green goodness!). This particular drink is fabulous if you're in a rush and haven't time to make a blended juice.

1 Put the powders in a cup and mix in a little of the juice to form a paste. Now gradually stir in the remaining liquids until blended.

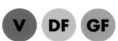

½ tsp spirulina powder

½ tsp chlorella powder

2 tsp [10 ml] aloe vera juice

generous 1 cup [250 ml] filtered water

Chai tea

Drink this when you need a recuperative cuppa; it's anti-inflammatory and antioxidant. I particularly like this spice mix, but add in any flavors you like, such as turmeric, ginger, cloves, even a few black peppercorns. **MAKES 4 CUPS**

1 Press the cardamom pods until they crack. Bring the water, tea, star anise, cinnamon, dates, and cardamom to a boil for three to five minutes until the tea is black and has reduced to about 1½ cups [350 ml]. Strain.

2 Add the nut milk and stir until hot. Place the used cardamom pods in the cups, if you want, for more flavor (but warn the drinkers!).

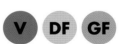

4 cardamom pods

1⅔ cups [400 ml] filtered water

4 to 5 black tea bags or
3 to 4 tsp loose leaf black tea

1 star anise

1 cinnamon stick

2 Medjool dates, pitted and chopped

1½ cups [350 ml] nut or Hemp milk
(see page 46)

Coconut milk

This deliciously smooth and alkalizing milk is youthing and versatile. Use it in curries, soups, ice creams, on breakfast cereals, or generally as a milk substitute. If you can get young coconuts it will taste even better. If you would like this milk less creamy, you can add more water. Or, if you want coconut cream, use less water. **MAKES ABOUT 4¼ CUPS [1 L]**

3 organic coconuts, to give 8¾ oz [250 g] coconut meat

1 Blend the coconut flesh with 4¼ cups [1 L] of filtered water for about three minutes. You can cover and store this for three days in the refrigerator, or freeze it in portions and take it out as you need.

Hemp milk

This milk is deeply nutritious, antioxidant, and high in anti-inflammatory omega-3s. It also has a great malty, nutty flavor that works very well on breakfast cereals or grains and in general cooking, but is a bit spooky in your tea or coffee! **MAKES ABOUT 4¼ CUPS [1 L]**

1½ cups [250 g] unhulled hemp seeds

2 tsp vanilla paste (optional)

1 The night before, soak the unhulled hemp seeds in plenty of filtered water. Let stand overnight to soften the hulls, then drain.

2 Put the hemp, 4¼ cups [1 L] of filtered water, and vanilla (if using) in a blender and whiz for about two minutes if you have a Vitamix (it could take a bit longer with a less powerful blender).

3 Place a nut bag or cheesecloth-lined strainer over a large bowl. Slowly pour the milk out of the blender, giving the cloth time to drain the liquid. Give the bag or cheesecloth a little squeeze to get out all the liquid. Cover and keep cold in the refrigerator. The hemp grinds can be given to the chickens, if you have them!

3

BREADS

"My doctor told me to stop having intimate dinners for four. Unless there are three other people,"

ORSON WELLES

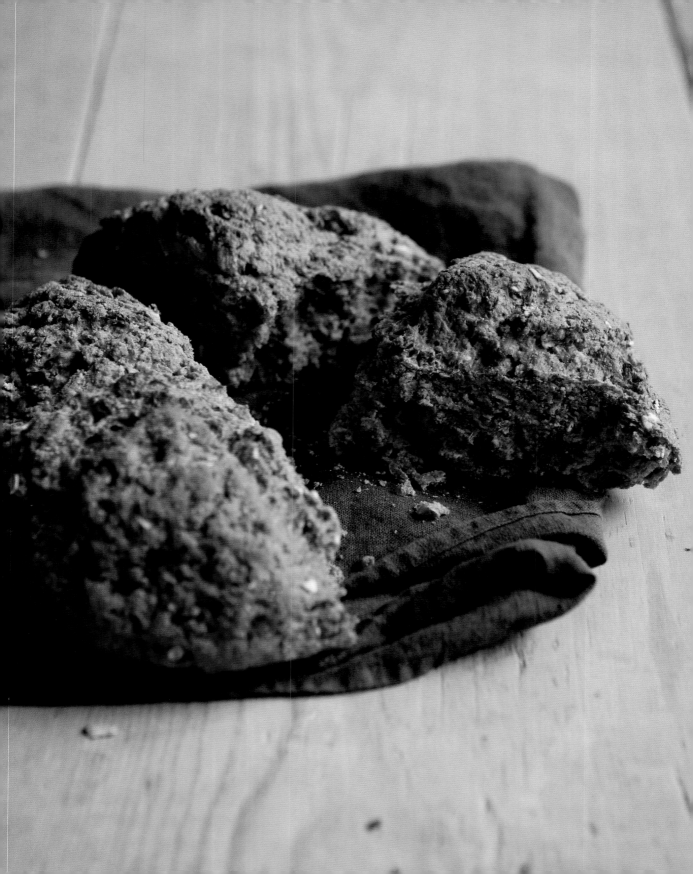

Butternut squash soda bread

Squash gives this rustic loaf a soft texture. Although not gluten-free, spelt is normally tolerated more easily by people who can't eat wheat. **MAKES 1 LARGE LOAF**

1 Preheat the oven to 425°F [220°C]. Roast the squash for 30 minutes, until soft, then mash and set aside to cool.

2 Mix the flour, oats, baking soda, and salt. Make a well in the center and add the squash and yogurt. Stir lightly until it just comes together.

3 Put on to a floured, nonstick baking sheet. Roughly form into a circle and make a cross on top with the handle of a wooden spoon.

4 Bake for 40 to 50 minutes, until golden and cooked. Serve warm or cool. This is especially delicious toasted.

14 oz [400 g] butternut squash, peeled, seeded, and coarsely chopped

3¾ cups [450 g] spelt flour, plus more to dust

½ cup [50 g] rolled oats

2 tsp baking soda

½ tsp Himalayan or Celtic salt

⅞ cup [200 g] plain yogurt

Banana bread

I call this a fast-track mood lift! Banana and vanilla both lift the spirits, while the cinnamon and the protein in the nuts help balance blood sugar, smoothing away any potential sugar-induced mood spikes engendered by the sweetness of the fruit …
MAKES 12 SLICES

1 Preheat the oven to 325°F [160°C]. Line the bottom and sides of a 2-lb [900-g] loaf pan with parchment paper, so it rises about ¾ in [2 cm] above the top of the pan edge.

2 Mash the bananas into a lumpy paste. Beat in the eggs, nut butter, and coconut oil until everything is well combined and fairly smooth. Fold in the remaining ingredients and immediately pour the batter into the prepared pan.

3 Transfer to the oven and bake for 1 to 1¼ hours, until golden and well risen, and a skewer inserted into the center comes out clean.

4 bananas

4 medium eggs, lightly beaten

5 Tbsp [75 g] nut butter, such as almond or cashew

3½ Tbsp [50 g] coconut oil, melted

scant 1 cup [75 g] ground almonds

scant ¼ cup [25 g] rice flour

1 tsp ground cinnamon

1 tsp gluten-free baking powder

½ cup [50 g] walnuts or pecans, coarsely chopped

1 tsp vanilla extract

pinch of Himalayan or Celtic salt

Gluten-free bagels

When I was a student in the USA I ate bagels every day and loved them. But when I gave up wheat and sugar, bagels were suddenly off the menu, so I had to come up with a youthing substitute pretty quickly. These are the closest I can get and (though I say it myself) they taste pretty darn good … **MAKES 6**

1 tsp fast-action yeast

1 tsp maple syrup (optional)

1⅔ cups [200 g] tapioca flour

½ cup [75 g] potato flour

½ cup [75 g] rice flour

2 tsp xanthan gum

pinch of Himalayan or Celtic salt

1 large egg, lightly beaten

1 tsp cider vinegar

1 tsp coconut oil

1 Sprinkle the yeast and maple syrup into a measuring cup and pour over 7 Tbsp [100 ml] of lukewarm filtered water. Stir to combine and set aside for five minutes, until the yeast is slightly frothy.

2 Meanwhile, sift the flours, xanthan gum, and salt into a large mixing bowl and make a well in the center. Pour in the frothy yeast mixture, the egg, cider vinegar, and coconut oil, with scant ¼ cup [50 ml] more lukewarm filtered water. Stir briskly to make a soft but not wet dough, adding a little more filtered water if it is dry. Knead the dough by hand or in a food mixer for five to 10 minutes, until smooth.

3 Roll the dough into six balls and flatten each slightly to make rounded disks. Make a hole in the center of each using your finger and widen it until it is about as large as a 50 cent piece. Cover the bagels with a damp dish towel.

4 Bring a large pan or stockpot of water to a boil and preheat the oven to 400°F [200°C].

5 Carefully slide two or three bagels at a time into the boiling water and simmer for one or two minutes, until they start to puff up slightly. Transfer to a nonstick baking sheet using a slotted spoon. Repeat with the remaining bagels.

6 Bake for 20 to 25 minutes, until golden and cooked through.

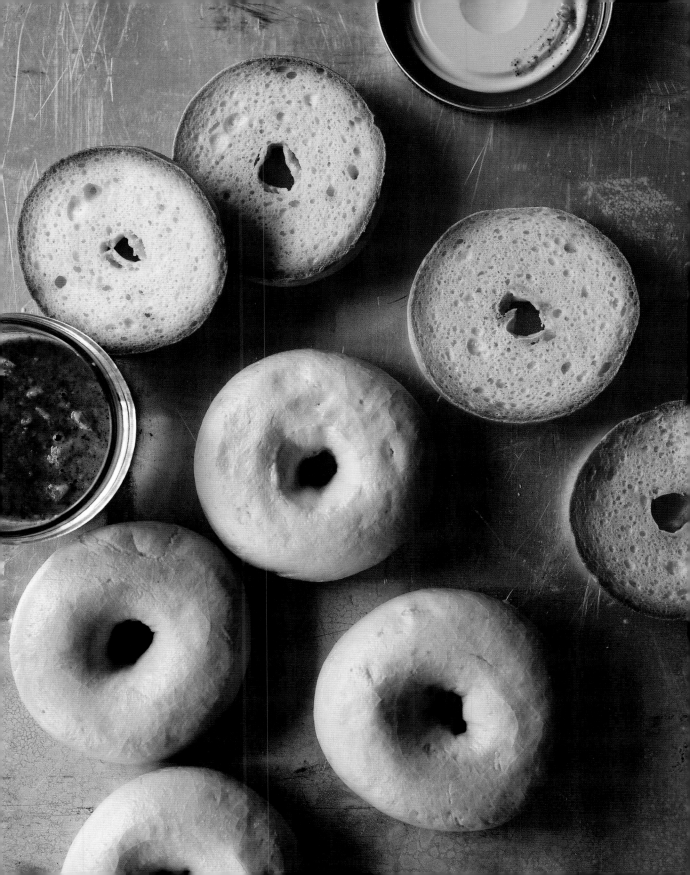

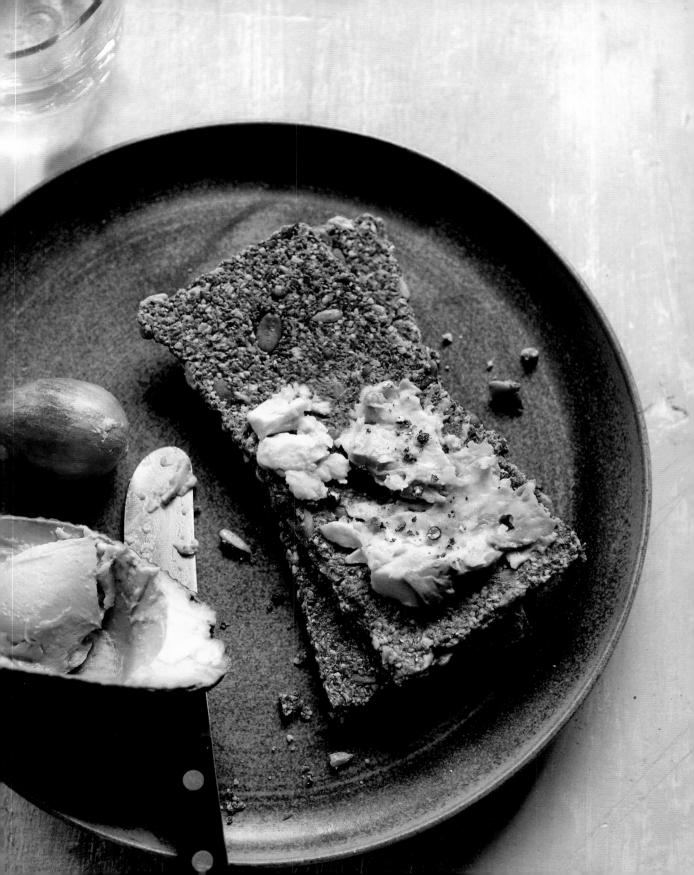

Mixed seed crackers

Easy and nutritious, packed with omegas and protein! These crackers are cooked at a low enough heat that they remain full of enzymes and goodness and can be eaten as part of a raw diet. Make them spicy or sweet as you like; they'll last for a week at room temperature (don't store them in the refrigerator, or they will lose their crunch). As you'll see in the rest of the book, I find them so versatile that I eat them with almost everything.

MAKES ABOUT 30

1 Preheat the oven to 250°F [120°C].

2 Mix all the seeds together in a bowl. If you would like some larger pieces in the crackers, take one-quarter of the seeds out. Grind the rest to a powder in a food processor or coffee grinder. Stir in the quinoa, oats, or coconut flour.

3 At this point decide whether you want the crackers spicy or sweet and add your chosen flavoring. The amount of flavor is up to you and you can experiment. If you like subtle tastes, add less, if you want something very savory or very sweet, add more. Return the whole seeds, if you took them out in the last step.

4 Gradually add generous 1 to 1¼ cups [250 to 300 ml] of filtered water while, with a wooden spoon or your hands, bringing the mixture together. It may need more filtered water to bind, so add accordingly. The mixture should come together like soft cookie dough.

5 Line a baking sheet with parchment paper. To help the paper lie flat, put some oil on the sheet and stick the parchment on top.

6 Put the dough on the baking sheet and roll it out thinly until it is about ¼ in (5 mm) deep. Score into equal squares or rectangles (this will make the crackers easier to break when cooked).

7 Place the sheet in the heated oven and let dry out for about an hour or until crisp. Don't be tempted to raise the oven temperature as this will brown the seeds and they will lose their nutritional value. Break along the scored lines and store in an airtight container.

FOR THE CRACKERS

1 cup [120 g] pumpkin seeds

¾ cup [120 g] flaxseeds

¾ cup [120 g] chia seeds

scant 1 cup [120 g] sunflower seeds

1⅓ cups [120 g] quinoa, oats, or coconut flour

a little coconut oil, for the sheet

FOR THE FLAVORINGS (CHOOSE FROM)

nigella seeds

red pepper flakes

cumin seeds

thyme leaves

rosemary leaves, minced

dates and/or unsulfured dried apricots, pitted and finely chopped

4

SOUPS

'The first wealth is health,

RALPH WALDO EMERSON

Gazpacho

Bursting with color and veggie goodness! Gazpacho is traditionally made with bread: here the gluten element has been replaced by cashews to add body as well as creaminess. This is an antioxidant and immune-booster; add a herb oil or pesto for more flavor. **SERVES 2 TO 3**

1 Finely chop the tomatoes, chile, and red bell pepper. Put the oil, vinegar, cucumber, garlic, and cashews in a blender and blend to a smooth, creamy consistency. Add all the other ingredients except the mint and blend for one or two seconds.

2 Chill in the refrigerator for a couple of hours, or serve immediately—depending on how cold you want the soup and how hot the day—poured into dishes and sprinkled with the mint.

3 tomatoes, quartered and seeded
1 red chile, seeded
1 red bell pepper, seeded
scant ¼ cup [50 ml] good virgin olive oil
2 Tbsp [35 ml] apple cider vinegar
1 cucumber, peeled
1 garlic clove, crushed
⅓ cup [50 g] cashews
1 Tbsp shredded mint leaves, to serve

Butternut and carrot soup

Carrots, sweet potato, and squash are all orange: a sign they contain youthing carotenes, which protect against cell damage. This creamy soup is rich in A and B vitamins, minerals, and tryptophan, which helps the production of feel-good hormone serotonin. **SERVES 4**

1 Preheat the oven to 400°F [200°C]. Roast the squash with the sweet potato and carrots for 15 minutes.

2 Add the coconut oil to a saucepan and gently fry the onion until translucent. Add the squash, sweet potato, carrots, and cumin and stir for one minute. Pour in the broth and bring to a simmer.

3 Continue to cook until the vegetables are soft. It should take about 10 minutes. Add the amino acids, nutritional yeast, and half the pine nuts and cook for another five minutes. Blend the soup in a blender, food processor, or with a handheld blender. Test for seasoning, adding a little pepper if you want.

4 Toast the remaining pine nuts in a dry frying pan. Pour the soup into bowls and sprinkle the pine nuts on top with the parsley, if using.

12 oz [350 g] butternut squash, peeled and chopped
1 sweet potato, peeled and chopped
5¼ oz [150 g] carrots, chopped
1 Tbsp coconut oil
1 onion, chopped
½ tsp ground cumin
3 cups [750 ml] vegetable broth, ideally homemade (see page 79)
15 drops of amino acids
2 large pinches of nutritional yeast
2 handfuls of pine nuts
freshly ground black pepper
small handful of chopped parsley leaves (optional)

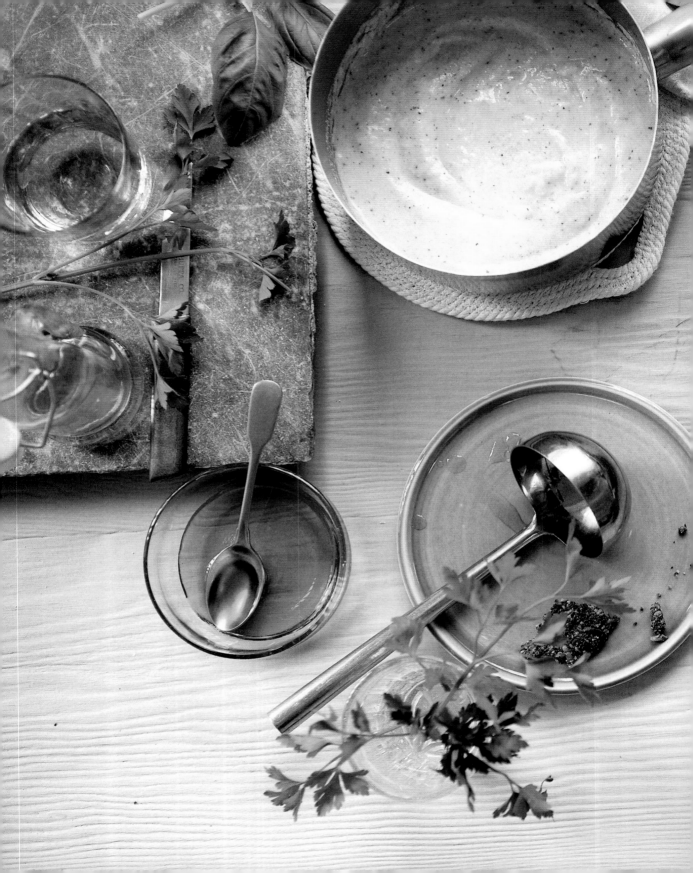

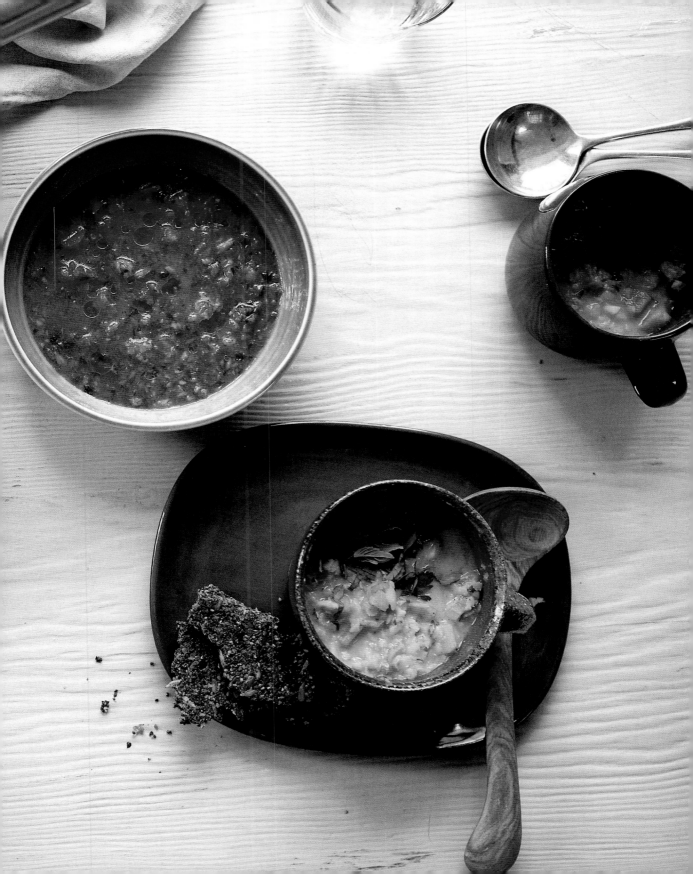

French onion soup

This ticks three youthing boxes—anti-inflammatory, antioxidant, digestive—and is great for detox, too. Eat it with Mixed seed crackers (see page 53), or make a "cheesy" crouton to go on top (use one of the cheese on toast recipes, see page 72, and trim to fit your bowl). **SERVES 2**

1 Steam-fry the onions with the coconut oil (see page 9), stirring frequently, until they begin to soften and caramelize. Be patient, as this will take at least 15 to 20 minutes.

2 Add the thyme, then pour in the broth. Bring to a boil, then reduce the heat to its lowest and simmer gently for another 10 minutes. Season to taste.

1½ onions, thinly sliced

1 tsp coconut or avocado oil

1 Tbsp thyme leaves

2½ cups [600 ml] vegetable broth, ideally homemade (see page 79)

pinch of Himalayan or Celtic salt

freshly ground black pepper

Spiced roast vegetable soup

Soup is a wonderful way of flooding your body with youthing vitamins, minerals, and herbs. This nutrient-rich soup is alkalizing, anti-inflammatory, easy on the digestion, and warms you up on a cold day. **SERVES 4 TO 6**

1 Preheat the oven to 425°F [220°C].

2 Toss the onion, carrots, and sweet potato in the coconut oil and roast for 25 to 30 minutes, until the vegetables have softened and are golden at the edges.

3 Sprinkle the ginger, garlic, and spices over the veg and stir through. Roast for another five minutes. Place in a blender with the hot broth and whiz until smooth. (Or place in a pan and blitz with a handheld blender.) Serve.

1 red onion, sliced

1½ lb [700 g] carrots, coarsely chopped

1 lb 2 oz [500 g] sweet potato, peeled and coarsely chopped

1 Tbsp coconut oil

1-in [2.5-cm] piece of gingerroot, grated

2 garlic cloves, crushed

2 tsp garam masala

½ tsp ground cumin

1 tsp ground turmeric

½ tsp black onion seeds

3 cups [750 ml] hot vegetable broth, ideally homemade (see page 79)

Versatile pea velouté

Yummy in a bowl, or even drizzled over poached eggs in the morning … Peas are high-fiber, low-cal, good for the heart, and full of antioxidants and anti-inflammatories. A legume, they are also high in protein, iron, calcium, and phosphorus. The most youthing way to eat this velouté is with another protein (that's your eggs), but it makes a tasty cold soup, too. **SERVES 2 TO 3, DEPENDING ON APPETITE AND HOW YOU USE IT**

1 In a sauté pan, gently steam-fry the shallots in the coconut oil (see page 9). Add the broth and peas and simmer until they are cooked.

2 Wilt the arugula in the pan with the peas for one minute, then put in a blender with the mint and salt and whiz until smooth. Use straightaway over egg dishes, or let cool, then chill, let down with a little filtered water to a consistency you prefer and eat it as a cold soup.

2 shallots, minced

1 tsp coconut oil

1¼ cups [300 ml] vegetable broth, ideally homemade (see page 79)

scant 2¼ cups [250 g] peas

1 oz [25 g] arugula (this will keep the soup a bright green)

2 Tbsp chopped mint leaves

pinch of Himalayan or Celtic salt

Versatile watercress velouté

A velouté variation which is nice in a bowl or used as a sauce with cold salmon … **SERVES 2 TO 4, DEPENDING ON APPETITE AND HOW YOU USE IT**

1 Heat the coconut oil in a large nonstick frying pan over medium-low heat and sauté the Iceberg and Boston lettuces for one to two minutes, until slightly softened.

2 Meanwhile, blanch the stems of the watercress and parsley in boiling filtered water for one minute, then add the watercress and parsley leaves, and blanch for another minute.

3 Transfer the lettuces, watercress, and parsley to a colander and drain over a bowl, setting aside the liquid, then plunge into ice-cold filtered water for five minutes. Drain, squeezing excess water from the leaves.

4 Blend the leaves, using the reserved cooking liquid, until you achieve your desired consistency. Push through a strainer before serving.

1 tsp coconut oil

½ Iceberg lettuce, shredded

1 Boston lettuce, shredded

3½ oz [100 g] watercress, stems removed and set aside

1 oz [30 g] parsley, stems removed and set aside

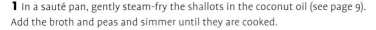
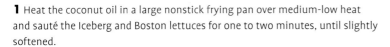

Nutty white soup

Try this when you need to alkalize. The coconut is high in potassium, magnesium, and caprylic acid, which can help the body overcome candida (see page 28). Anti-inflammatory and a good immune-booster, whack in some garlic if you're feeling under the weather. **SERVES 6**

1 Steam-fry the onion and celery (see page 9) in the coconut oil and a little filtered water for two minutes, then add the leeks and continue for another five minutes. Then stir in the ground almonds.

2 Take from the heat and gradually stir in the coconut cream, then the broth. Return to the heat and add the bouquet garni and lemon zest. Simmer for about 10 minutes until all the vegetables are soft.

3 Season with the yeast flakes and pepper, then let sit for 10 minutes to let the flavors combine. Take out the bouquet garni and blend the soup in a blender or food processor, or with a handheld blender, until smooth. Reheat if necessary. You can pour a little coconut cream on top of the served soup, if you want, then sprinkle with chopped parsley for color.

1 onion, chopped

1 head of celery, trimmed and sliced

2 Tbsp coconut oil

3 leeks, sliced (about 14 oz/400 g)

scant 1 cup [75 g] ground almonds

scant ¼ cup [50 ml] coconut cream, plus more to serve (optional)

3 cups [750 ml] vegetable broth, ideally homemade (see page 79)

1 bouquet garni

finely grated zest of 1 unwaxed lemon

3 tsp nutritional yeast flakes

freshly ground black pepper

small handful of chopped parsley leaves

Red lentil and cashew soup

The long list of ingredients looks daunting, but this high-protein soup is a youthing treasure; try it out! It's good if you're detoxing or want something nutritious but light. SERVES 6

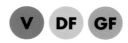

1 Melt the oil in a heavy pan and add the celery, butternut squash, garlic, onion, carrot, and bay leaves. Fry until the vegetables are tender.

2 Add the lentils, tomatoes, vinegar, cumin, and nutmeg, stir, then pour in the broth. Bring to a boil and simmer, adding the thyme and parsley. Drain and finely chop the cashews and add them, too.

3 Simmer until the lentils are nice and soft; you may have to add a bit more liquid if it gets too thick. When cooked and the thickness of light cream, take off the stove, stir, cover, and let sit for a few hours, or chill until later.

4 When ready to serve, either put the whole soup in a blender (don't forget to remove the bay leaves), or leave it chunky. Reheat gently, add the basil, if using, and adjust the seasoning.

4 tsp [20 g] coconut oil

1 celery stalk, finely sliced

4 oz [110 g] butternut squash, peeled, seeded, and finely chopped

2 garlic cloves, minced

1 onion, minced

1 small carrot, finely chopped

2 bay leaves

1 cup [180 g] red lentils

2 large tomatoes, seeded and chopped

scant ¼ cup [50 ml] cider vinegar

1 tsp ground cumin

½ tsp freshly grated nutmeg

3 cups [700 ml] vegetable broth, ideally homemade (see page 79)

1 Tbsp thyme leaves

1 Tbsp chopped parsley leaves

scant ½ cup [65 g] cashews, soaked in filtered water overnight

1 Tbsp shredded basil leaves (optional)

freshly ground black pepper

5

SALADS

'To eat is a necessity, but to eat intelligently is an art.'

FRANÇOIS DE LA ROCHEFOUCAULD

Aromatic mackerel and fennel salad

Fennel is yummy with mackerel; it gives a tart, anise riposte to the oiliness of the fish and brings a whole lot more youthing benefits, too, as it's an inflammation- and cancer-fighter and is also supersoothing for the digestion. **SERVES 4**

1 Soak the fennel seeds in warm filtered water for two hours. Drain.

2 Put the soaked, drained fennel seeds in a pan and dry-fry for two or three minutes, or until lightly toasted. Set aside to cool. Slice the fennel as finely as possible, on a mandolin if you have one.

3 Mix together the fennel slices, olive oil, and lime juice in a large bowl until combined, then set aside to marinate for 30 minutes.

4 Meanwhile, for the mackerel, place the coriander seeds and shallot with the peppercorns in a sauté pan, pour in 7 Tbsp [100 ml] of filtered water, and bring to a simmer. Tip in the lemon slices, then place the mackerel in the pan and cover.

5 Let the mackerel steam-fry (see page 9) until the water has evaporated and the fish is cooked. There is enough fat in the mackerel to keep the dish moist, there is no need to add extra oil.

6 Add half the cooled, toasted fennel seeds to the fennel salad with the arugula and mix again to combine.

7 To serve, divide the fennel salad equally among four serving plates. Place one fillet of mackerel on each and spoon the salad dressing around the edge of the plates. Scatter over the remaining toasted fennel seeds.

FOR THE FENNEL SALAD

1 tsp fennel seeds

½ fennel bulb, trimmed

4 tsp [20 ml] olive oil

1 tsp lime juice

½ oz [15 g] wild arugula

FOR THE MACKEREL

¼ tsp coriander seeds, toasted and crushed

1 banana shallot, thinly sliced

½ tsp pink peppercorns, crushed

½ lemon, sliced

4 mackerel fillets, pin-bones removed, skin scored (ask your fish supplier to do this)

stalks from a 1-oz [25-g] package of cilantro

Barley salad with figs and arugula

Barley is an underused, undervalued grain, but it's a great weapon in your youthing armory. It helps control blood sugar, reduces cholesterol, and visceral fat (the health-damaging stuff that wraps around your internal organs). It is low-cal yet leaves you feeling fuller for longer. This salad is a combination of delicious, digestive, antioxidant, and alkalizing … how youthing is that? **SERVES 2**

½ cup [100 g] pearl barley

4 fresh figs, quartered

1¾ oz [50 g] arugula leaves

2 scallions, sliced

leaves from a small bunch of Italian parsley or cilantro, coarsely chopped

¼ cup [30 g] almonds, coarsely chopped

juice of 1 lemon

2 tsp extra virgin olive oil

1¾ oz [50 g] feta cheese, or ½ avocado (optional)

1 Tip the pearl barley into a strainer and rinse well under cold filtered water to remove the excess starch. Pour into a pan and cover with cold filtered water. Bring to a boil, cover, and simmer over medium-low heat for 40 to 50 minutes, until tender but with a slight bite. Drain and run under cold filtered water until cool. Drain once more. Set aside in a large salad bowl.

2 Combine the figs, arugula, scallions, herbs, and almonds with the barley. Toss through the lemon juice and oil, then crumble over the feta or slice over the avocado, depending which you are using.

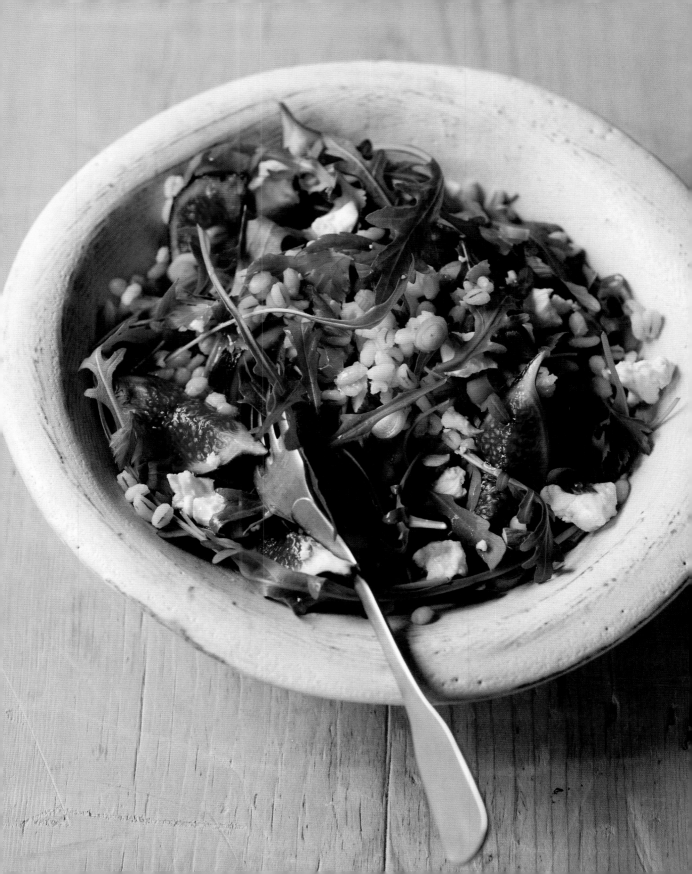

Salad bouquet

A wonderful way to make alkalizing greens look hip and artsy. Youthing salad greens help digestion, work as detoxifiers, and are slimming and nutritious. I've specified the leaves and herbs I prefer, but choose a mixture of them, depending how you want it. **SERVES 2**

1 Pick up half the Chinese leaves (as the largest, they should be on the outside of your bouquet). Take out any large stalks. Hold them in your left hand (if you are right-handed) and add leaves individually inside them, until it begins to look like a flower arrangement.

2 When half of all the leaves have been added, wrap the large Chinese leaves around it so the bouquet is finished. Cut the bottom so the stems are the same length (don't cut it so short that you can't tie it). Meanwhile, put the scallion strips into boiling water. Use the scallion as a "string" to secure the bouquet around its stalks.

3 Take two or three carrot and zucchini strips and lay on a counter next to each other, slightly overlapping to form a band. Wrap into a circle and stand it up on a plate. Place the salad bouquet inside; the band should keep it in place. Repeat to form a second bouquet.

8 large Chinese leaves

handful each of watercress, spinach, radicchio, and lettuce leaves

5 basil leaves, 5 mint leaves, and a handful of parsley leaves

a few fennel fronds

6 scallions, cut lengthwise into strips (to use as "string")

1 carrot, cut into long slices with a mandolin or potato peeler

1 zucchini, cut into long slices with a mandolin or potato peeler

Waldorf salad with mayonnaise

A delicious sweet-and-sour combination with a big walnut bite. This is a light, alkalizing, well-balanced dish; the sweetness of the pear is offset nicely by the protein in the raw egg and nuts, ensuring the sugars are slowly released. **SERVES 4**

1 Make the mayonnaise as directed on page 82.

2 To make the salad, toss all the ingredients except the mayonnaise together and sprinkle over the lemon juice. Stir in 2 to 3 Tbsp of the mayonnaise and serve. The remaining mayonnaise can be kept in an airtight container in the refrigerator for two or three days.

1 quantity Mayonnaise (see page 82)

2 firm pears, sliced

4 celery stalks, chopped

¾ cup [75 g] walnuts, coarsely chopped

3½ oz [100 g] arugula leaves

juice of ½ lemon

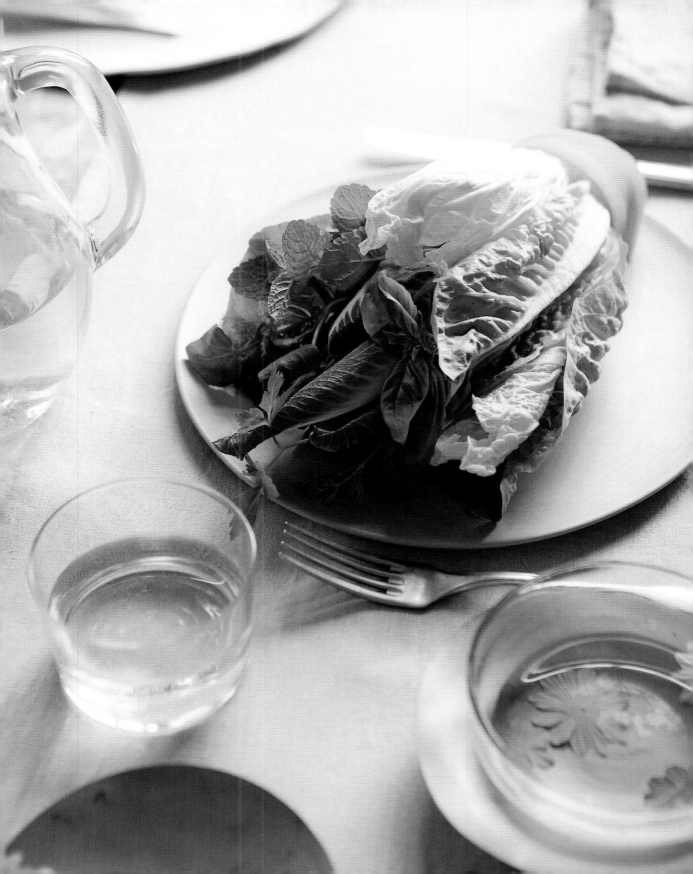

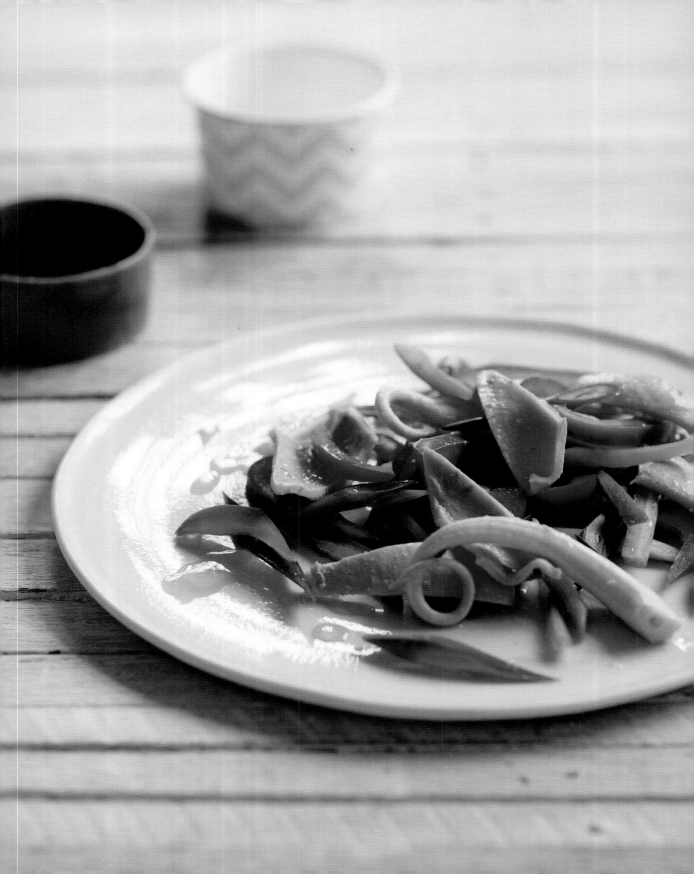

Octopus salad

People think octopus is difficult to get right, but doing it this way is easy: you simply let it simmer and wait. It's worth it for the taste and it's a cheap deal, too, as an octopus feeds many people. This salad is high in vitamins, minerals, and omegas and low in saturated fat and calories. A good dinner party appetizer, or eat it as your protein over a week. Scale up the amount of salad to serve more people. **MAKES ABOUT 10 SERVINGS**

1 The octopus tentacles and body can be eaten, but first remove all the dirt from the suckers. This takes a bit of time, but it is important that it is clean. Also clean the head.

2 Put all the ingredients to cook the octopus into a large pot of filtered water filled to the top, add the octopus, and simmer for three hours. The amount of flavorings is really down to personal taste. I rather like having a strong taste, so I would put in rather a large amount of each.

3 You will find the skin of the octopus comes off easily. Cut the tentacles off and then take off the suckers and skin. Slice into pieces and marinate the octopus in the olive oil and lemon for several hours.

4 When ready to serve the octopus, slice the peppers and celery into strips and then chop at an angle to create 1-in [2.5-cm] slices with angled tops and bottoms. Chop the scallions.

5 Place the salad vegetables on a plate, spoon over the octopus and its marinade, and serve.

TO COOK THE OCTOPUS

4½ lb [2 kg] octopus

1 large onion, chopped

3 celery stalks, chopped

1 lemon, halved

10 thin slices of gingerroot

⅓ oz [10 g] sprigs of rosemary

⅓ oz [10 g] sprigs of thyme

⅓ oz [10 g] sprigs of basil

1 lemon grass stalk, bruised

7 Tbsp [100 ml] white wine vinegar

TO MARINATE THE OCTOPUS

scant ¼ cup [50 ml] olive oil

juice of 1 lemon

FOR THE SALAD (SERVES 2)

¼ green bell pepper

¼ red bell pepper

¼ celery stalk

2 scallions

6

SNACKS

'Eating crappy food isn't a reward— it's a punishment,

DREW CAREY

Youthing nut bar

This was a favorite in my last book, so we put it in again! It is a fabulous snack when you're on the move, plus it tastes miles better (and I would bet it is also better for you) than any store-bought health bar. It's nutritionally well-balanced and, at the same time, satisfyingly sweet. **MAKES 6**

1 To make the sweet apricot paste, put the apricots in a bowl and pour boiling filtered water over to cover. Leave for one minute, drain, then place in a bowl with the orange juice and ⅝ cup [150 ml] filtered water and let soak for two or three hours until the apricots are plumped up. Blend the mixture with the ground seeds.

2 For the tahini mixture, bring a pan of filtered water to a boil. Drop in the apricots and blanch for one minute, then drain. Chop finely and mix with all the remaining ingredients.

3 Preheat the oven to 350°F [180°C].

4 Put the oats, almonds, sesame, sunflower, and pumpkin seeds on a baking sheet in the oven and roast lightly for 10 minutes. Remove from the oven. Thoroughly mix the warmed oat mixture with the tahini mixture, then spread evenly in an 8-in [20-cm] deep-sided nonstick baking pan. Let cool in the refrigerator.

5 If you want a treat, you can add a chocolate topping to the bars. First melt the chocolate in a heatproof bowl over a pan of simmering water (the bowl should not touch the water). Then spread on top of the nut bar with a hot palette knife or the back of a spoon. Let set in the refrigerator, then chop into squares.

6 The bars will keep in an airtight container in the refrigerator for 10 days. Or freeze them in freezer bags, so you always have some handy.

FOR THE SWEET APRICOT PASTE

⅔ cup [110 g] dried unsulfured apricots

⅝ cup [150 g] fresh orange juice

2 to 4 Tbsp ground hemp or flaxseeds

FOR THE TAHINI MIXTURE

⅔ cup [110 g] dried unsulfured apricots

scant ½ cup [200 g] gluten-free tahini

8 oz [220 g] Sweet apricot paste (see above)

⅓ cup [50 g] mixed almonds and sunflower seeds, ground together finely

FOR THE BARS

1¼ cups [110 g] oats

⅓ cup [50 g] whole almonds, chopped

4 Tbsp [50 g] sesame seeds

⅓ cup [50 g] sunflower seeds

scant ½ cup [50 g] pumpkin seeds

3½ oz [100 g] 80% cocoa solids vegan semisweet chocolate (optional)

Vegan "cheese" and tomato toastie

If you suffer from salty cheese cravings, this neat toastie is your salvation! Simple and filling, it's also nicely youthing thanks to the cashews (high in vitamins, minerals, and good omega fatty acids) and vitamin B12-rich nutritional yeast which soothes the nervous system and helps you feel bouncy and alive. **SERVES 1**

1 Toast the bread lightly on both sides. Spread on the cheese and top with the slices of tomato.

2 Place under the broiler for about five minutes until the tomato starts to cook and the cheese bubbles.

3 Serve hot with Sweet tomato relish (see page 84).

1 slice of sprouted spelt bread, or bread of choice

about 2 Tbsp Creamy "cheese" (see page 81)

1 tomato, finely sliced

"Cheese" on toast with basil and olive oil

Sprouted bread contains more protein and fewer carbs than bread made from conventional grain. This version of the ever-popular cheese on toast is gorgeously gooey but also fabulously tangy, thanks to the basil. **SERVES 1**

1 Toast the bread lightly on both sides. Spread on the cheese and top with the shredded basil.

2 Drizzle with oil and place under the broiler for about five minutes until the cheese bubbles and turns golden brown. Serve hot.

1 slice of sprouted spelt bread, or bread of choice

about 2 Tbsp Creamy "cheese" (see page 81)

a couple of basil leaves, shredded

drizzle of avocado oil

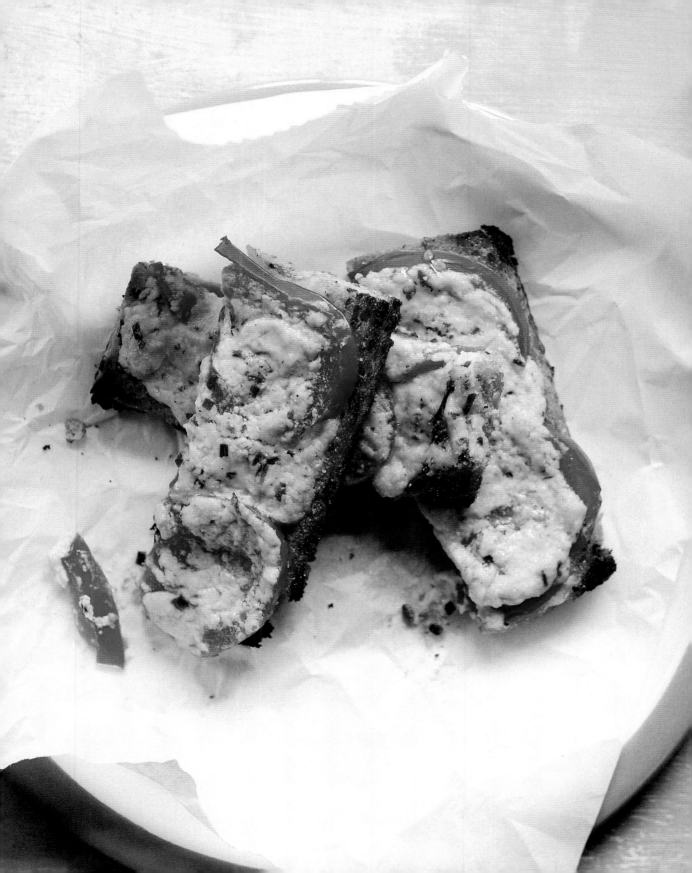

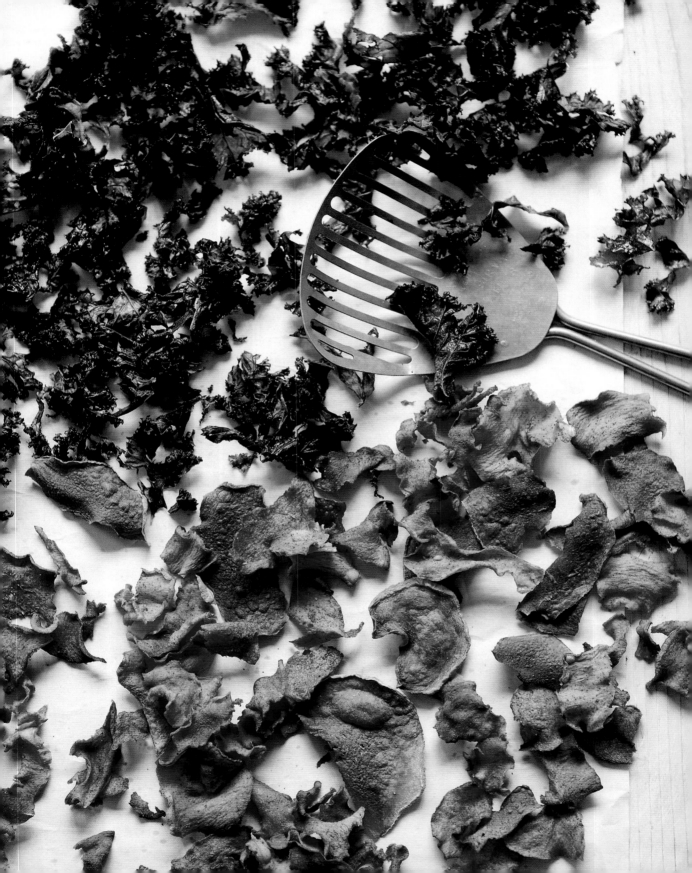

"Cheesy" kale chips

You can buy kale chips everywhere now, but nothing beats making them yourself: not only do they taste better, but you know what's in them! If the "cheesy" flavor doesn't do it for you, try cayenne pepper or fennel seeds in place of the nutritional yeast. **SERVES 4**

3½ oz [100 g] kale, washed, thoroughly dried, and cut into bite-size pieces

2 tsp coconut oil, melted

2 Tbsp nutritional yeast flakes

1 Preheat the oven to 350°F [180°C]. Toss the kale in the oil and yeast flakes until well coated. Spread out on a baking sheet and bake for 15 to 20 minutes, turning over every so often, until crisp and golden at the edges.

2 These are great as a snack, or used as a healthy alternative to croutons on soup. Store in an airtight container for up to three days.

Butternut squash chips

I love the taste of potato chips, but have not eaten a bag for more than 15 years. These homemade chips are a versatile substitute, just change the spices when you want a different taste. Butternut squash is low in calories but high in antioxidants, folic acid, and minerals, which are good for metabolism and the endocrine system. So eat up! **SERVES 2**

3½ oz [100 g] butternut squash, peeled and seeded

1 tsp coconut oil, melted

pinch of ground cinnamon

pinch of Himalayan or Celtic salt

1 Preheat the oven to 275°F [140°F].

2 Line a large baking sheet with parchment paper. Slice the squash very finely with a knife or a mandolin and toss with the oil, cinnamon, and salt to coat.

3 Spread the slices evenly on the baking sheet, being careful not to overlap them, and bake in the oven for 20 to 30 minutes, turning halfway through, until crisp and golden. If some of the slices crisp up before others, remove them from the oven and set aside on a wire rack lined with parchment paper to cool.

Popcorn with seaweed salad

I love watching movies but never touch the popcorn offered in movie theaters. This tastes much better than the synthetic offering, plus it is nutritionally sound and low calorie. It's great at any time, plus children love it, too. **MAKES 1 LARGE BOWL, OR 2 PORTIONS**

1 Tbsp [15 g] coconut oil

½ cup [100 g] organic popping corn

1 large handful of dried seaweed salad, or more if you like

1 to 2 tsp Himalayan or Celtic salt if needed

1 Gently melt half the coconut oil in a heavy pan, then increase the heat to high. Sprinkle in the corn and cover. Reduce the heat a little so the popcorn does not burn. As soon as you hear the corn popping, gently shake the pan. When the popping has stopped, take off the heat and pour into a bowl.

2 Melt the rest of the oil and toss in the handful of seaweed, more if you require, and stir. Sprinkle it over the popcorn. Taste and see if you want to add the salt as well (the seaweed is very salty) and add (or not) to taste. Serve immediately.

Chia tabbouleh

Tabbouleh is the easiest way of getting your greens. It goes with anything, or you can eat it in mounds on its own. Parsley is one of the most youthing plants around, said to be so high in vitamin K and calcium that if you eat a handful a day it will ward off thinning of the bones. **SERVES 2**

3⅓ cups [100 g] Italian parsley leaves

generous 1 cup [30 g] mint leaves

2 tomatoes, finely chopped

½ cucumber, finely chopped

4 scallions, minced

1 Tbsp olive oil

juice of 1 lemon

¼ tsp sumac

1 Tbsp chia seeds

1 Mince the parsley and mint with a sharp knife so as not to bruise the herbs. Transfer to a mixing bowl and toss with the tomatoes, cucumber, scallions, olive oil, and lemon juice.

2 Sprinkle over the sumac and chia seeds just before serving.

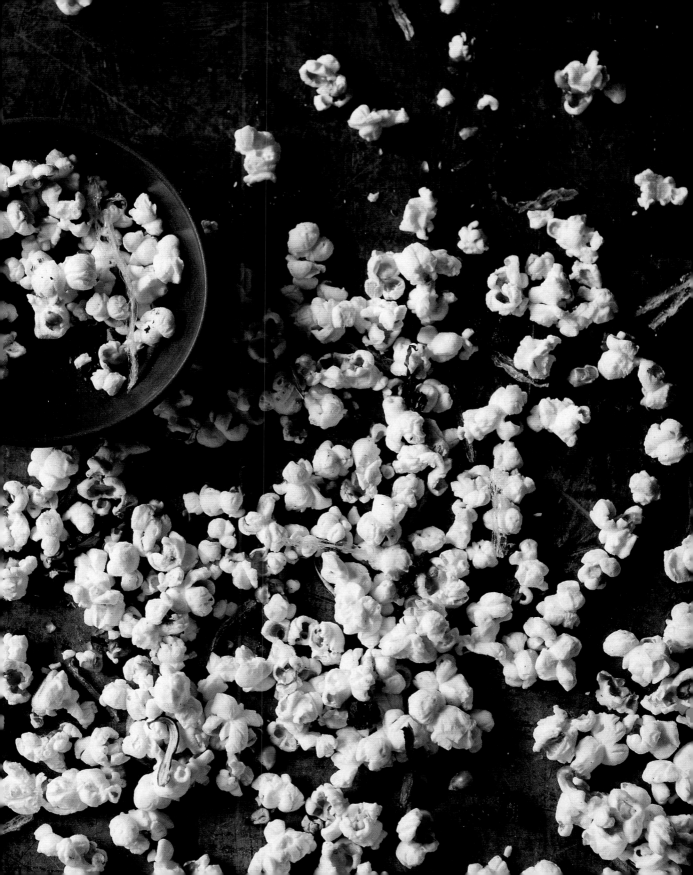

7

SAUCES AND ACCOMPANIMENTS

'You are what what you eat eats,

MICHAEL POLLAN

Vegetable broth

Using homemade broth in recipes is a fabulous way of getting minerals and vitamins … while making dishes taste delicious. It is low in sodium and high in nutrition. The kombu seaweed here ensures this most youthing stock helps your thyroid function and keeps your weight in control, too. **MAKES 6½ to 8½ CUPS** [1.5 to 2 L]

1 Place all the ingredients in a heavy pan with 5.2 quarts [6 L] of filtered water and bring to a boil.

2 Reduce the heat and let simmer, uncovered, for 50 minutes to one hour. It will reduce to about one-third of its original volume.

3 Strain, leave to cool and use as necessary, or store in the refrigerator for up to three days, or freeze it in portion-sized batches.

2 carrots, peeled and chopped

½ head of celery, chopped

2 onions, peeled and halved

¼ turnip, peeled and chopped

1 parsnip, peeled and halved

1 leek, trimmed and halved

6 cabbage leaves

small bunch of parsley stalks

4 black peppercorns

1 star anise

1 slice of orange

4 strips of kombu seaweed

1 slice of red bell pepper

3 bay leaves

Fish broth

White fish bones make the most delicious, nourishing, mineral-rich broth. Drink this for breakfast if you need a boost, or use it in fish dishes. **MAKES ABOUT 3½ CUPS** [800 ML]

1 Add the carrot, celery, ginger, and vinegar to a heavy pan. Let the mix dry-fry and then add the fish bones. When the bones have fried a bit (but not too much), add 4¼ cups [1 L] of filtered water.

2 Add the bay leaves, peppercorns, thyme, and parsley, depending on the taste you want.

3 Bring to a boil, then reduce the heat and simmer for 20 minutes for a light taste. If you want a stronger taste, cook for another 10 minutes, but no more. Remove the foam as it bubbles to the top.

4 When it is ready, pour into a bowl through a colander. This keeps in the refrigerator for a couple of days, or freeze it in portion-sized batches.

1¾ oz [50 g] carrot, peeled and chopped

1¾ oz [50 g] celery, chopped

1¾ oz [50 g] piece of gingeroot, chopped

7 Tbsp [100 ml] cider vinegar

14 oz [400 g] fish bones from white fish

3 bay leaves

6 black peppercorns

bunch of thyme, to taste

bunch of parsley, to taste

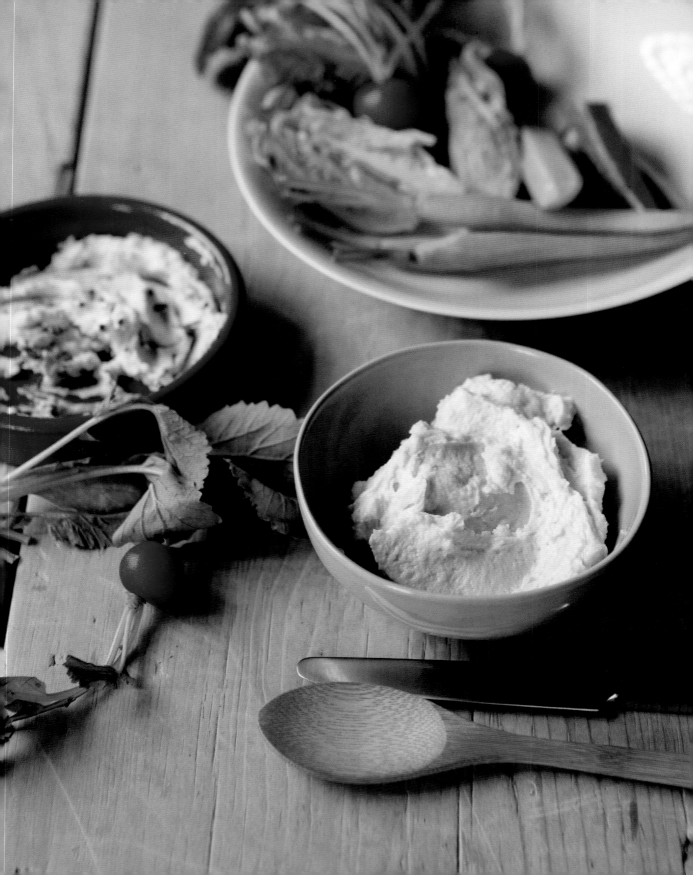

Creamy "cheese"

The guilt-free snack of the moment, as far as I am concerned. Deliciously indulgent and creamy-cheesy, this is full of omegas and alkalizing benefits. **SERVES 2**

1 Soak the cashews in a bowl of plentiful filtered water for two to three hours. Drain.

2 Blend the cashews, garlic, lemon juice, and vinegar with ¼ cup (60 ml) of filtered water, then measure the liquid and keep a note of the volume. Transfer to a small pan and sprinkle with the agar flakes, using 1 Tbsp of flakes per one cup [250 ml] of liquid. Heat through and simmer, stirring gently, for two to three minutes, then add the melted coconut oil. Stir in the parsley and chives now, if you like, and add the salt, if you think it needs it.

3 Pour into a small glass bowl and put into the refrigerator for two to three hours before serving, sprinkled with the herbs if you didn't add them earlier. Serve with bagels, salads, and crudités.

scant ½ cup [65 g] cashews

1 garlic clove, coarsely chopped

juice of ½ lemon

2 tsp cider vinegar

agar flakes (amount depends on volume of liquid)

1 Tbsp coconut oil, melted

1 Tbsp minced parsley leaves

1 Tbsp chopped chives

½ tsp Himalayan or Celtic salt (optional)

Walnut "Parmesan"

Another dairy-free "cheese"; sprinkle on salads, pasta, and rice dishes as you would Parmesan, or it's fabulous in stuffed baked tomatoes (see page 130). **MAKES 2 OZ [55 G]**

1 Put all the ingredients in a food processor and whiz to finely chop.

2 Scrape into a small bowl and chill for two to three hours before serving.

½ cup [55 g] walnuts

3 Tbsp nutritional yeast flakes

1½ pinches of Himalayan or Celtic salt

Mayonnaise

This creamy mayonnaise tastes better than anything you could buy in a store and you know you're getting nutritious, youthing ingredients. The raw egg protein is easily absorbed by the body, the good omega oils are anti-inflammatory, it's high in healing vitamin E, and good for joints, brain, and heart. When it comes to the egg here, the fresher the better. **MAKES 5¼ OZ [150 G] SERVES 6**

1 egg yolk

1 small garlic clove, crushed

pinch of Himalayan or Celtic salt

juice of ½ lemon

7 Tbsp [100 ml] light olive oil

scant ¼ cup [50 ml] canola oil

freshly ground black pepper

1 Drop the egg yolk, garlic, salt, and a few drops of the lemon juice into a mixing bowl and whisk briefly to blend. Add 1 tsp of one of the oils and whisk until the mixture is well combined. Add another 1 tsp and whisk until the mixture is really thick. At this point, gradually pour in both the oils in a very thin stream while whisking. If the mixture begins to split, add a little lemon juice or a splash of filtered water.

2 Keep adding the oil and whisking until you have a thick, rich mayonnaise, then season to taste with lemon juice and pepper. If the consistency is too thick, stir in a little more filtered water.

Almond butter

Almonds are a nutritionally very well-balanced mix of protein, fiber, good omega fats, and carbohydrate and they help hair, nails, and skin look young and radiant. **MAKES ABOUT 4½ OZ [130 G]**

1¾ cups [145 g] leftover almond grounds (if you are making almond milk), or 1¾ cups [145 g] ground almonds

2 Tbsp gluten-free tahini, plus more if needed

2 dates, pitted

1 Put all the ingredients in a blender and pulse until smooth; add more tahini if the mixture is too dry.

2 Serve on sprouted toast, eat with crudités, or add to olive oil to make an almond vinaigrette.

Turmeric marinade

Turmeric is one of my favorite spices, good for pretty much everything and a great anti-inflammatory (I even give it to my dog for her arthritis!). But how to get it down you in quantity, as it turns everything yellow and tastes rather strong? This marinade is a great way to do it and jazz up your fish at the same time. You can also use a bit of it in a broth for a stew or curry.

SERVES 4

1 Blend all the ingredients except the basil into a paste. Tear up the basil finely and stir through the paste.

2 Use as a marinade for white fish: cover pieces of fish with it in a nonreactive container, turning to coat, then cover and refrigerate it for up to 12 hours, turning occasionally.

1 Tbsp chopped gingerroot

1 Tbsp chopped celery

1 Tbsp chopped parsley leaves

1 Tbsp lemon juice

1 Tbsp olive oil

2 tsp ground turmeric

1 tsp minced garlic or onion

3 basil leaves

Tomato jellies

If you are bored with tomato sauce, this is a funky way to add highly concentrated tomatoes to a soup or cooked dish (just drop a few jellies in). You can even spread a jelly on a Mixed seed cracker (see page 53)! I eat large quantities of tomatoes for the lycopene; it can help to prevent lines and wrinkles in the skin. **MAKES ABOUT 1 ICE-CUBE TRAY FULL (2 CUPS/500 ML)**

5 tomatoes

1 red bell pepper

2 pinches of nutritional yeast flakes

freshly ground black pepper

juice of 1 lemon

2 Tbsp agar flakes

finely sliced basil leaves (optional)

1 Quarter and seed the tomatoes and pepper and put them in the blender. Blend until very smooth. Measure the liquid; it should be two cups [500 ml], if not, add filtered water until it is.

2 Put the liquid into a small pan and stir in the yeast flakes, pepper, and lemon juice. Sprinkle the agar flakes on the top. Slowly bring to a boil, stirring occasionally. Reduce the heat and simmer for about three minutes, then let cool slightly. Stir in the basil (if using), then pour into an ice-cube tray.

3 Place in the refrigerator. It will take 20 to 30 minutes to set.

Sweet tomato relish

Use this delicious, versatile relish on veggie burgers, cheese on toast, or with salads. It is alkalizing and full of antioxidants. The garlic, chile, and shallot boost the immune system, too. This is a fresh relish, so cannot be potted and kept for weeks, but it shouldn't be a problem to eat it up quickly. **SERVES 4**

1 garlic clove

1 banana shallot

1 tsp coconut oil

2 tomatoes, peeled (see page 119) and chopped

¼ tsp minced mild red chile

2 Tbsp cider vinegar

1 Tbsp tamarind pulp

1 Mince the garlic and shallot and steam-fry in the oil (see page 9) until translucent. Add the tomatoes and chile and stir to combine. Add the cider vinegar and tamarind with 3 Tbsp of filtered water. Let the relish reduce over gentle heat until the tomatoes have taken on a jamlike consistency.

2 Remove from the heat and cool. This can be eaten hot or cold.

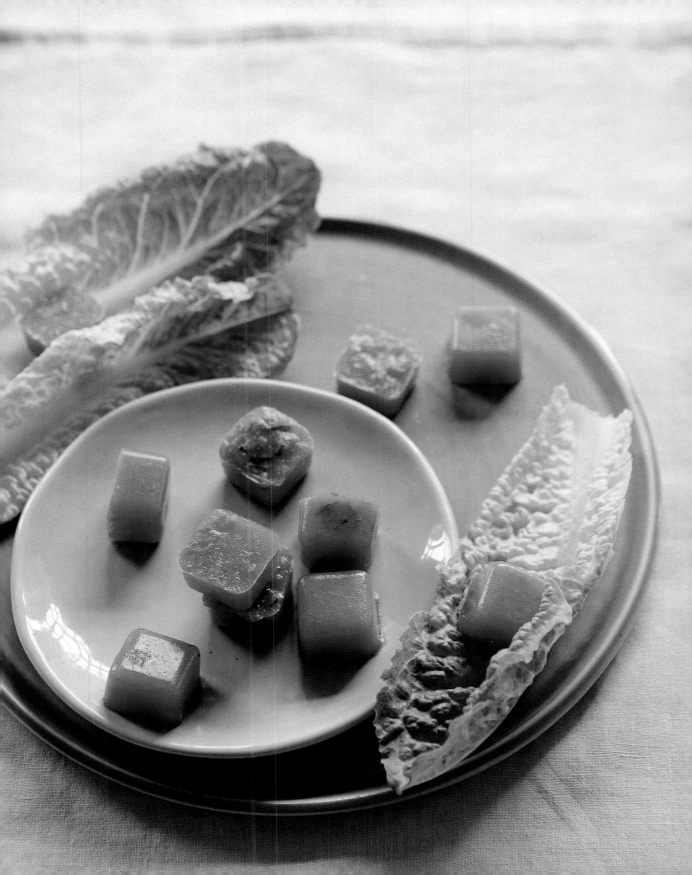

8

APPETIZERS

'Start by doing what's necessary;
then do what is possible; and
suddenly you are doing
the impossible,

FRANCIS OF ASSISI

I offer recipes for a few sushi-style rolls wrapped in seaweed in this chapter. Seaweed is a great functional youthing food, it grows in salt water, and contains an almost identical range of minerals to those used by the human body. Especially rich in calcium and iodine—which controls metabolism and helps the body copy with stress—seaweed also contains anti-inflammatory factors and other plant compounds that are thought to offer protection against aging diseases including cancer. It may also help you lose weight and burn any unhealthy fat stored around your middle.

People are often frightened of cooking seaweed, because they aren't used to handling or eating it. So here are a few ideas to help you create interesting and youthing appetizers …

Avocado, cauliflower, and spicy tofu nori rolls

"Nori" is the Japanese word for red edible seaweed. It is usually dried into thin sheets and used to roll fish or vegetables. This spicy, nutrient-dense appetizer will keep you fuller for longer, thanks to avocado's heart-healthy fats. **MAKES 12**

½ head of cauliflower

½ avocado, flesh chopped

1 Tbsp cider vinegar

2 nori sheets

⅜-in [1-cm] slice of gingerroot, peeled and finely sliced

3½ oz [100 g] firm gluten-free tofu, sliced into matchsticks

1 Tbsp coarsely chopped cilantro leaves

¼ tsp red pepper flakes (optional)

2-in [5-cm] piece of cucumber, sliced into matchsticks

¼ red bell pepper, sliced into matchsticks

1 Cut the cauliflower into florets and steam for six to eight minutes, until tender. Cool and dry in the steamer for a few minutes before pulsing in a food processor until the cauliflower resembles rice. Add the avocado and pulse a few more times until combined. Transfer to a mixing bowl and stir in the vinegar. Cool.

2 Lay a nori sheet out on a sushi rolling mat and spoon over half the cauliflower "rice." Spread the rice over the nori, leaving a ¾-in [2-cm] gap along the edge furthest from you. Lay half the ginger, tofu, cilantro, pepper flakes, cucumber, and pepper in an even horizontal line across the center of the rice (along its length) and carefully roll the nori up tightly away from you using the mat, to form a cylinder. Roll in plastic wrap and chill until required. Repeat with the remaining nori sheet and filling. Cut each into six equal rolls with a very sharp knife, to serve.

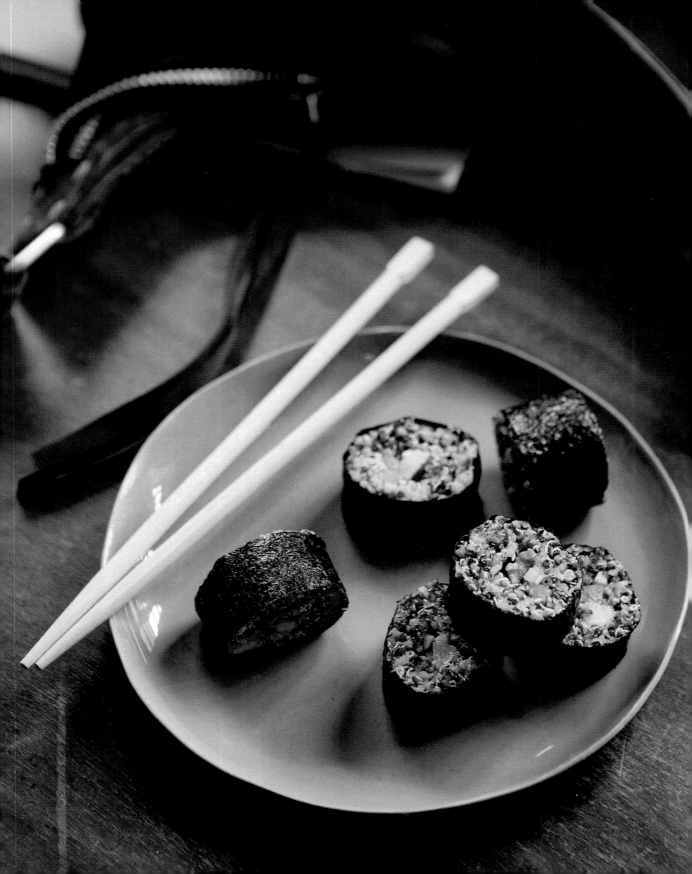

Quinoa maki rolls

Quinoa is a great alternative to rice; it is gluten-free, high in protein, fiber, antioxidants, and must-have minerals including magnesium, manganese, and copper. These are tasty, filling, and youthing rolls. **MAKES 24**

1 Peel and pit the avocado, finely slice the flesh, and sprinkle with the lime juice, tossing gently to coat to prevent discoloration.

2 Cook the quinoa in boiling water for eight to 10 minutes, until softened but still with a little bite. Drain. Sprinkle over the vinegar, stir it in evenly (and add the wasabi if you want, though you can add it to the filling), and set aside while you prepare the other ingredients.

3 When the quinoa is completely cool, lay a sheet of nori out on a sushi rolling mat or cutting board with a long edge facing you. Spoon one-quarter of the quinoa onto the sheet and spread out, leaving a ¾-in [2-cm] gap along the edge furthest from you. Lay out one-quarter of the pepper, ginger, cucumber, carrot, and avocado in a line across the center of the nori sheet (along its length) and spoon over ¼ tsp wasabi paste, if you didn't mix it into the quinoa earlier.

4 Roll the sheet up tightly away from you, using the mat to help, to form a cylinder. Roll in plastic wrap and chill until required. Repeat with the remaining nori sheets and filling. Cut each into six equal rolls with a very sharp knife, to serve. Serve with a dish of tamari, or wasabi, or both, if you like, for dipping.

1 avocado

juice of ½ lime

⅓ cup [75 g] quinoa

2 tsp cider vinegar

1 tsp wasabi paste, plus more to serve (optional)

4 nori sheets

1 red bell pepper, finely sliced

⅜-in [1-cm] slice of gingerroot, peeled and finely sliced

2-in [5-cm] piece of cucumber, sliced into matchsticks

1 small carrot, peeled and sliced into matchsticks

gluten-free tamari, to serve (optional)

Cauliflower maki rolls

I eat these to destress or when I need an energy kick; the iodine in the seaweed helps with low thyroid function and low energy and is alkalizing, too. Cauliflower is a very underrated vegetable: It is detoxifying and low-cal yet tastes like carbs, so you can get what feels like a carb fix without topsy-turvy-ing your blood sugar. **MAKES 12**

1 Peel and pit the avocado, finely slice the flesh, and sprinkle with the lime juice, tossing gently to coat to prevent discoloration.

2 Cut the cauliflower into florets and steam for six to eight minutes, until tender. Let cool and dry in the steamer for a few minutes before pulsing in a food processor until the cauliflower resembles rice. Transfer to a mixing bowl and stir in the vinegar. Set aside until completely cool.

3 Lay a nori sheet out on a sushi rolling mat and spoon over half the cauliflower "rice." Spread it over the nori, leaving a ¾-in [2-cm] gap along the edge furthest from you. Lay half the avocado, ginger, chives, cucumber, carrot, and pepper in an even horizontal line across the center of the rice (along its length) and carefully roll the nori up tightly away from you using the mat, to form a cylinder. Roll in plastic wrap and chill until required. Repeat with the remaining nori sheet and filling. Cut each into six equal rolls with a very sharp knife, to serve.

½ avocado

1 tsp lime juice

½ head of cauliflower

1 Tbsp cider vinegar

2 nori sheets

⅜-in [1-cm] slice of gingerroot, peeled and finely sliced

12 chives

2-in [5-cm] piece of cucumber, sliced into matchsticks

1-in [2.5-cm] piece of carrot, peeled and sliced into matchsticks

¼ red bell pepper, sliced into matchsticks

Mackerel pâté

This is such a youthing treat, anti-inflammatory, and with a double dose of good fats, it tastes deliciously rich and creamy. Eat with Mixed seed crackers (see page 53) or toast, or with a green or tomato salad for a quick and easy appetizer. **SERVES 2**

1 To cook the mackerel, first remove the skin as it is easier to cook.

2 Pour scant ¼ cup [50 ml] of filtered water into a heavy frying pan and lay in the mackerel fillets. Let cook, turning occasionally. As the water runs dry, add a little more to fill the bottom of the pan. Cooking in this way means that the mackerel holds all its oil and is much more moist. It should take three or four minutes to cook.

3 When it is ready, take the mackerel off the heat and, when it has cooled, check for bones by breaking up the mackerel in your fingers.

4 Skin and pit the avocado and mash the flesh into the mackerel with the onion (if using). Add lemon juice to taste and the sumac and mash some more, either by hand, or blend for a smoother texture. Add black pepper to taste. Scrape into a bowl and serve, or chill for a few hours first.

2 mackerel fillets, about 4¼ oz [125 g] each

1 avocado, about 3½ oz [100 g]

¼ onion, finely sliced (optional)

juice of 1 lemon, or to taste

1 tsp sumac

freshly ground black pepper

Avocado mousse wrapped in spinach

This is the perfect dinner party appetizer: Easy to make, it looks and tastes a million dollars, and is supergood for you. (Just scale up the quantities to make more.) Guests will feel sated but "light" as the happy fats in the avocado work their magic alongside four great alkalizers and detoxers: Spinach (high in vitamin K and calcium); watercress; arugula; and fennel. As a protein option, goat cheese is easier to digest than other dairy products, but leave it out if anyone is lactose-intolerant. **SERVES 2**

1 Brush two ramekins with oil and line the bottoms with wax paper or parchment paper.

2 Drop the spinach leaves into boiling water, then immediately drain and plunge them into a bowl of cold water. When they are cold, drain once more and pat dry.

3 Spread the spinach leaves out and use them to line the ramekins, with excess overhanging the top (to cover the mousse later).

4 Place the peeled, pitted avocado, basil, goat cheese, chia seeds, scallion, parsley, lime juice, and nutmeg in a blender with 1 Tbsp of filtered water. Pulse-blend until smooth.

5 Spoon the avocado mousse into the ramekins and cover the top with the overhanging spinach. Refrigerate for two or three hours.

6 Put the salad ingredients in a bowl. To make the dressing, put all the ingredients into a jar, screw on the lid, then shake to emulsify. Toss the dressing with the salad and place on two plates.

7 Tip each ramekin upside down onto a board; the mousse will tip out. Remove the papers and place on the salad. Finish with Mixed seed crackers (see page 53) to serve alongside the mousse, if you like.

GF

FOR THE MOUSSE

a little olive oil

8 large spinach leaves

1 large avocado

8 basil leaves

scant ¼ cup [40 g] soft goat cheese

1 tsp chia seeds

1 scallion, finely sliced

2 sprigs of Italian parsley

juice of ½ lime

pinch of freshly grated nutmeg

Mixed seed crackers (see page 53), to serve (optional)

FOR THE SALAD

handful of mixed arugula and watercress leaves

½ sweet pepper, sliced into matchsticks

8 green beans, sliced into matchsticks

FOR THE DRESSING

2 Tbsp hemp oil

1 Tbsp lime juice

large pinch of ground fennel seeds

freshly ground black pepper

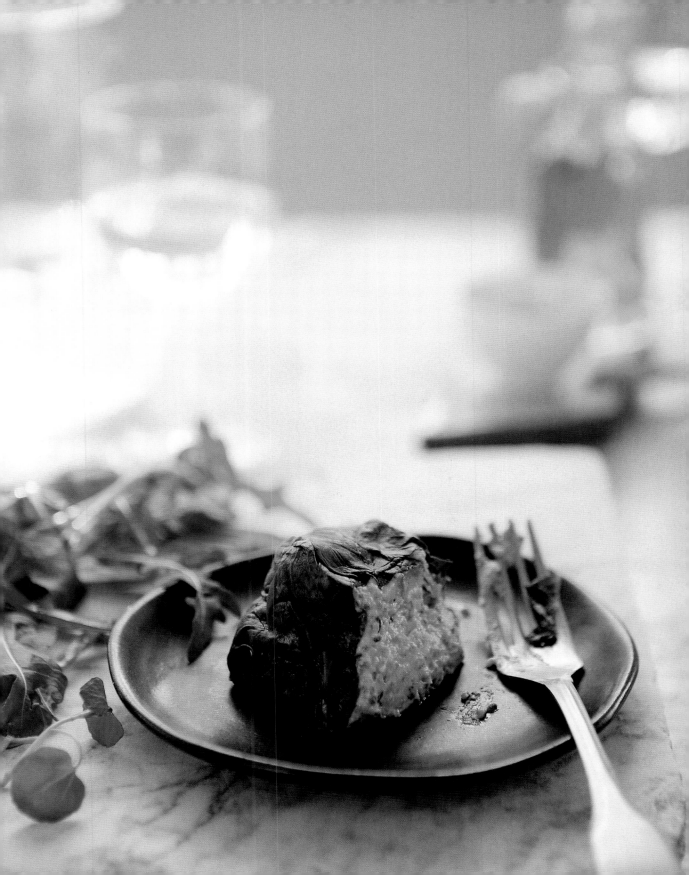

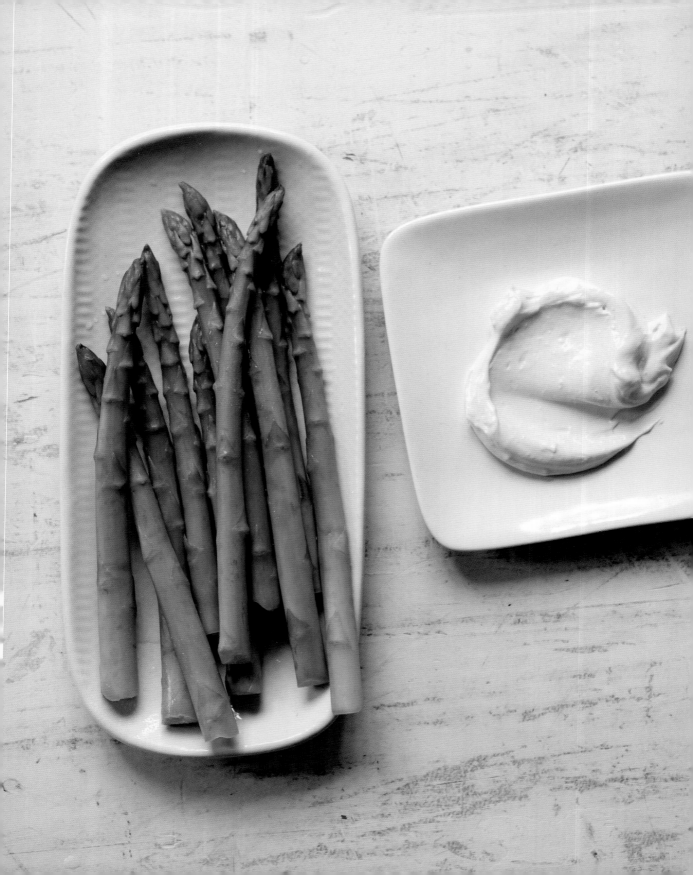

Asparagus with homemade mayonnaise

Asparagus, said Marcel Proust, "transforms my chamber-pot into a flask of perfume." Need I say more? It has a short season, but is worth the wait. You can make asparagus into a soup, add it to salads, or just indulge in the lovely spears with some mayonnaise, as I do here. **SERVES 4 TO 6 AS AN APPETIZER**

1 to 2 bunches of asparagus, as required

1 quantity Mayonnaise (see page 82)

1 Place filtered water in the bottom half of a steamer pan or asparagus steamer and bring to a boil.

2 Trim the dry ends off the asparagus. If the spears are thick, peel the thickest parts lightly with a vegetable peeler. Place them in the steamer. Steam for five to 10 minutes depending on the thickness of the asparagus, or until tender.

3 When ready, drain well. Serve with homemade Mayonnaise (see page 82).

9

MAIN MEALS

'Perfection is not attainable,
but if we chase perfection we can
catch excellence,

VINCE LOMBARDI

Moroccan spicy lentil stew

A delicious, densely nutritious meal; lentils are without doubt among the best sources of vegetable protein. The herbs and spices here fire up the digestion and are also anti-inflammatory and immune-boosting. **SERVES 6**

1 Heat the oil in a large sauté pan or Dutch oven over medium-low heat. Fry the onion for about five minutes, until softened. Add the garlic and all the ground spices and fry for another two minutes, until fragrant.

2 Stir in the sweet potatoes and lentils and cover with the vegetable broth. Simmer, stirring occasionally, for 20 minutes. Stir in the tomatoes and zucchini. Simmer for another 10 to 15 minutes, until the lentils are tender.

3 Serve sprinkled with the cilantro and lemon juice.

2 tsp avocado oil

1 large onion, chopped

4 garlic cloves, crushed

1 tsp ground cumin

1 tsp ground coriander

1 tsp ground turmeric

½ tsp ground cinnamon

1 tsp sweet paprika

8¾ oz [250 g] sweet potatoes, peeled and chopped

½ cup [100 g] Puy lentils

3 cups [750 ml] vegetable broth, ideally homemade (see page 79)

4 large tomatoes, chopped

8¾ oz [250 g] zucchini, chopped

handful of cilantro, coarsely chopped

2 Tbsp lemon juice

Crustless roast vegetable tart

This taste bud sensation is a great anti-inflammatory and immune booster and is high in protein, minerals, and antioxidants. I serve it at girlfriend lunches (we swoon as it cooks, the smell is so enticing), because it works for vegetarians, the gluten-free 'n' all. **SERVES 6**

1 Preheat the oven to 400°F [200°F]. Lightly oil a 9-in [23-cm] ovenproof dish with a little of the coconut oil.

2 Place the peppers and tomatoes in a roasting tray and drizzle over the remaining oil. Stir in the garlic, tomato paste, thyme, turmeric, and cumin and roast in the oven for 15 to 20 minutes, until the vegetables are softened and nicely roasted. Remove from the oven and set aside.

3 Sift the flour into a mixing bowl and make a well in the center. Crack the eggs into the well and pour in half the almond milk. Beat the mixture with a whisk until smooth, then gradually beat in the remaining milk and ⅝ cup [150 ml] of filtered water to make a batter. Stir through the roasted vegetables, followed by the nutritional yeast flakes, lemon zest, parsley, and red pepper flakes (if using).

4 Pour the mixture into the prepared dish and bake for 20 to 30 minutes, until set and golden. Let rest for 10 minutes, then slice and serve hot or cold.

2 tsp coconut oil, melted

2 red bell peppers, sliced

8¾ oz [250 g] cherry tomatoes

2 garlic cloves, crushed

1 Tbsp tomato paste, or boiled-down tomatoes

1 tsp thyme leaves

½ tsp ground turmeric

½ tsp ground cumin

scant 2 cups [175 g] gram flour

3 large eggs

2 cups [500 ml] almond milk

2 Tbsp nutritional yeast flakes

finely grated zest of 1 unwaxed lemon

2 Tbsp chopped Italian parsley leaves

½ tsp red pepper flakes (optional)

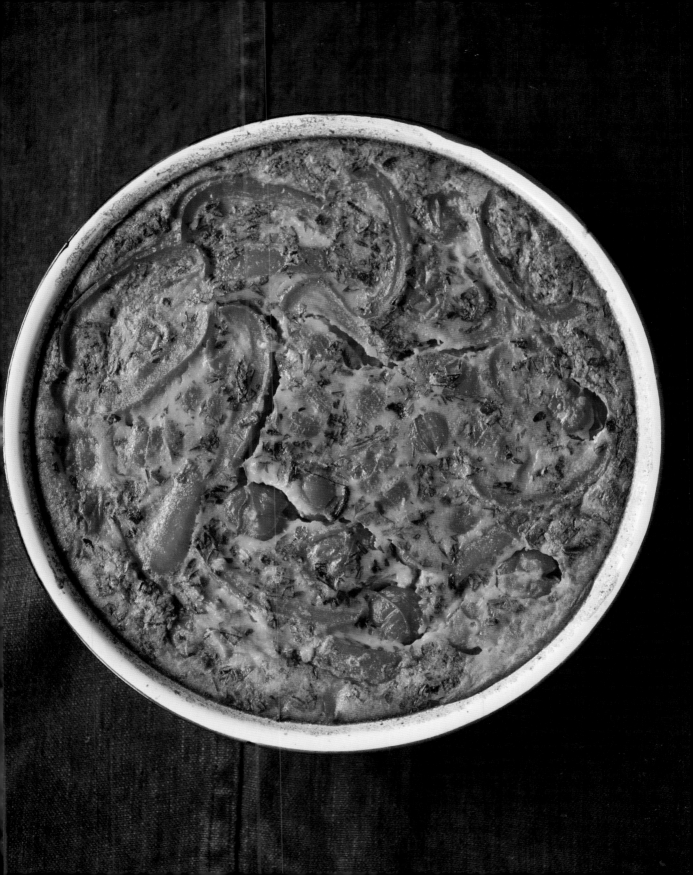

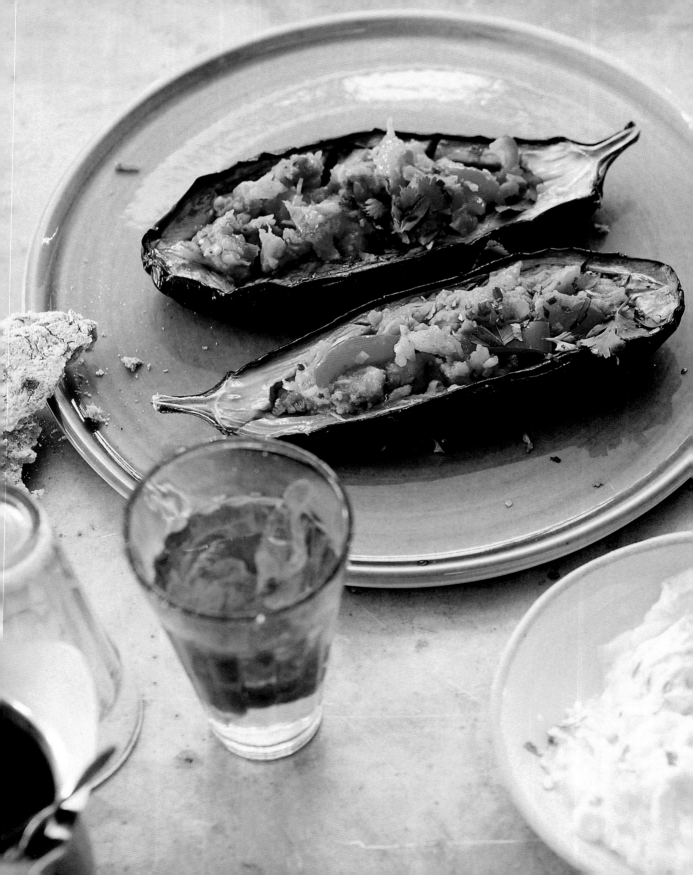

Turkish stuffed eggplants with tzatziki and spelt flatbreads

This is for people who love cooking and have time to do it! It makes an exotic, supertasty dinner party centerpiece while still being therapeutic: Anti-inflammatory, an aid to digestion, and thoroughly filling. **SERVES 4**

1 To make the stuffed eggplants, preheat the oven to 425°F [220°C]. Cut each eggplant in half lengthwise. Score the cut flesh in a crisscross pattern and lay, scored-side up, on a baking sheet. Drizzle the eggplants with half the oil and transfer to the hot oven for 20 to 30 minutes, until they are soft and burnished. Scoop most of the flesh out of the eggplants and set aside.

2 Heat the remaining oil in a large, nonstick frying pan over medium-low heat and add the onion. Fry gently, adding a little filtered water as necessary if the onion looks as if it may catch, until softened. Add the peppers and fry for another two minutes, then add the garlic, spices, and salt. Fry for another minute or two, until fragrant, then finally add the tomatoes and scooped-out eggplant flesh. Increase the heat and simmer for five minutes or so, until cooked through and fairly thick. Add a little filtered water to let down if necessary. Spoon the tomato mixture into the empty eggplant skins and return to the oven for five to eight minutes, until browned and bubbling hot.

3 Meanwhile, make the tzatziki and flatbreads. For the tzatziki, spoon the yogurt into a bowl and grate in the cucumber. Stir in the garlic and mint and add lemon juice to taste.

4 To make the flatbreads, sift the flour into a mixing bowl and stir in the remaining dry ingredients. Make a well in the center and add the oil and enough warm filtered water (up to ⅞ cup/200 ml) to make a fairly stiff dough. Bring the dough together with your hands—adding a little more filtered water if necessary—and knead briefly. Divide the dough into four and roll each piece out on a lightly floured counter to a ¼ in [5 mm] thickness. Heat a large, nonstick pan over high heat and dry-fry the flatbreads one by one, until puffed up and slightly charred.

5 Serve the eggplants scattered with parsley, lemon juice, and red pepper flakes (if using) alongside the tzatziki and flatbreads.

FOR THE EGGPLANTS

4 medium-small eggplants

2 to 3 tsp coconut oil, melted

1 medium onion, finely sliced

4 red bell peppers, sliced

2 fat garlic cloves, crushed

2 tsp cumin seeds

½ tsp ground cinnamon

½ tsp ground turmeric

pinch of Himalayan or Celtic salt

8 medium tomatoes, chopped

handful of Italian parsley leaves, chopped

squeeze of lemon juice

pinch of red pepper flakes (optional)

FOR THE TZATZIKI

¾ cup [175 g] goat or sheep yogurt

½ cucumber, peeled and seeded

1 small garlic clove, crushed

2 Tbsp chopped mint leaves

juice of ½ lemon, or to taste

FOR THE SPELT FLATBREADS

1⅔ cups [200 g] whole grain spelt flour, plus more to dust

pinch of Himalayan or Celtic salt

2 tsp dukkah, or ras el hanout

1 tsp baking powder

1 tsp avocado or coconut oil

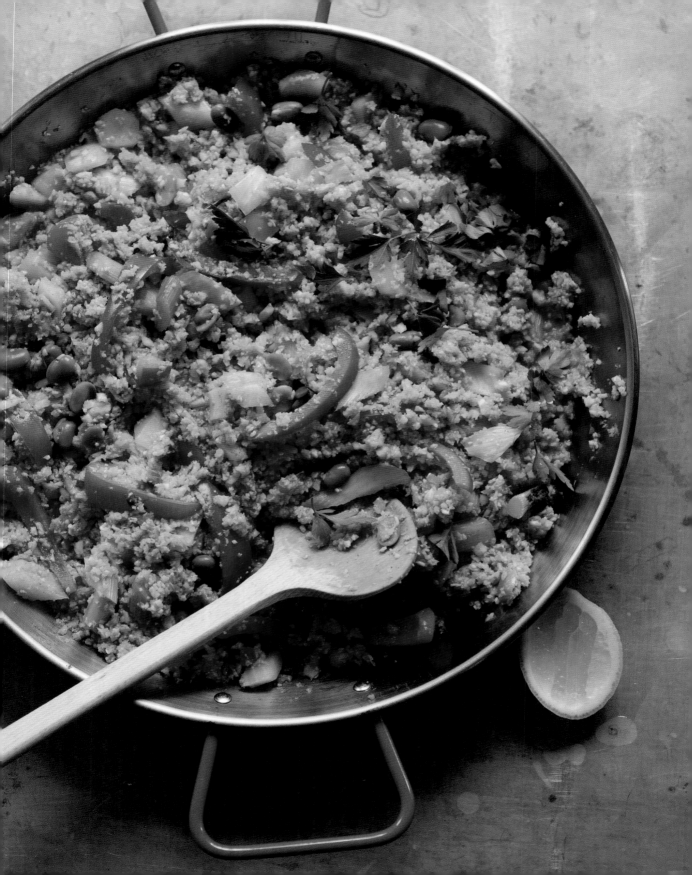

Cauliflower and vegetable paella

This is a great youthing option for a light supper or a lazy night in. It's tasty and low in calories. **SERVES 4**

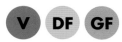

1 Pulse the cauliflower florets in a food processor until they resemble grains of rice.

2 Heat the oil in a large sauté or medium paella pan over medium-low heat. Add the onion and gently fry, adding a little water if it begins to dry out, until softened. Add the fennel and peppers and fry for two minutes, until beginning to color. Add the garlic, paprika, and turmeric and fry for another minute, until fragrant. Stir through the cauliflower rice until combined and pour in enough broth to cover. Sprinkle over the saffron, cover, and simmer for five to eight minutes, or until the broth has been mostly absorbed and cauliflower is tender. Add more broth if necessary.

3 Tip in the fava beans and cover for another minute or two until tender. Stir in the parsley and lemon juice and serve immediately.

1 medium cauliflower, cut into florets

2 tsp coconut oil

1 onion, minced

1 small fennel bulb, coarsely chopped

2 red bell peppers, sliced

2 garlic cloves, crushed

2 tsp sweet paprika

1 tsp ground turmeric

2 cups [500 ml] vegetable broth, ideally homemade (see page 79), plus more if needed

pinch of saffron strands

7 oz [200 g] fava beans

handful of Italian parsley leaves, coarsely chopped

juice of ½ lemon

Gardener's pie

Unlike shepherd's pie (lamb) or cottage pie (beef), this vegan, dairy-, and gluten-free version of the traditional dish is made from the best produce of the garden. It has a deep gravy taste you'll love on a cold winter's day, while the powerful nutrients in the root veg will give you energy and vigor. **SERVES 6**

1 Steam-fry the onion (see page 9) with a little filtered water and the coconut oil, add the carrot, eggplant, and garlic, and fry for two to three minutes. Reduce the heat and cook until the veg are a little soft.

2 Quarter and seed the tomatoes and blend the flesh. Add half to the veg with the thyme, parsley, and a good pinch of caraway. Stir gently, then add the beans, broth, and miso paste. Cook slowly, stirring occasionally, for about 10 minutes. Be careful it doesn't catch on the pan and, if you think it might, add a splash more filtered water. Now add the nutritional yeast flakes, the amino acids, and the rest of the tomato. Put into a pie dish.

3 Preheat the oven to 400°F [200°C].

4 Now prepare the topping. Boil both types of potato together until tender, then drain and mash with the nutritional yeast flakes, amino acids, and broth, seasoning with pepper. Spread the potato on top of the filling, fluff the top with a fork, then bake for 20 minutes.

NOTE
You can of course use dried pinto or aduki beans, that you have soaked and cooked yourself. When cooked, they will weigh almost double their dried weight.

FOR THE FILLING

½ onion, chopped

½ tsp coconut oil

1 carrot, chopped

¼ eggplant, chopped

1 garlic clove, minced

3 tomatoes

2 tsp thyme leaves

1 Tbsp chopped parsley leaves

pinch of caraway seeds

14-oz [400-g] can of pinto or aduki beans, drained and rinsed

¼ cup [60 ml] vegetable broth, ideally homemade (see page 79)

½ tsp gluten-free miso paste

2 tsp nutritional yeast flakes

10 drops of liquid amino acids

FOR THE TOPPING

2 sweet potatoes

1 medium mealy potato

1 tsp nutritional yeast flakes

10 drops of liquid amino acids

scant ¼ cup [50 ml] vegetable broth, ideally homemade (see page 79)

freshly ground black pepper

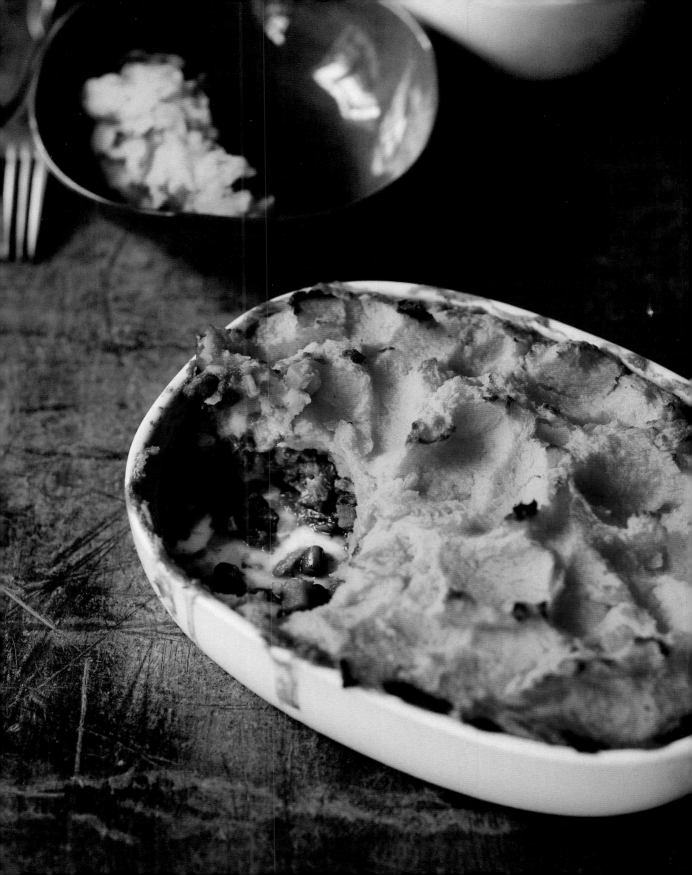

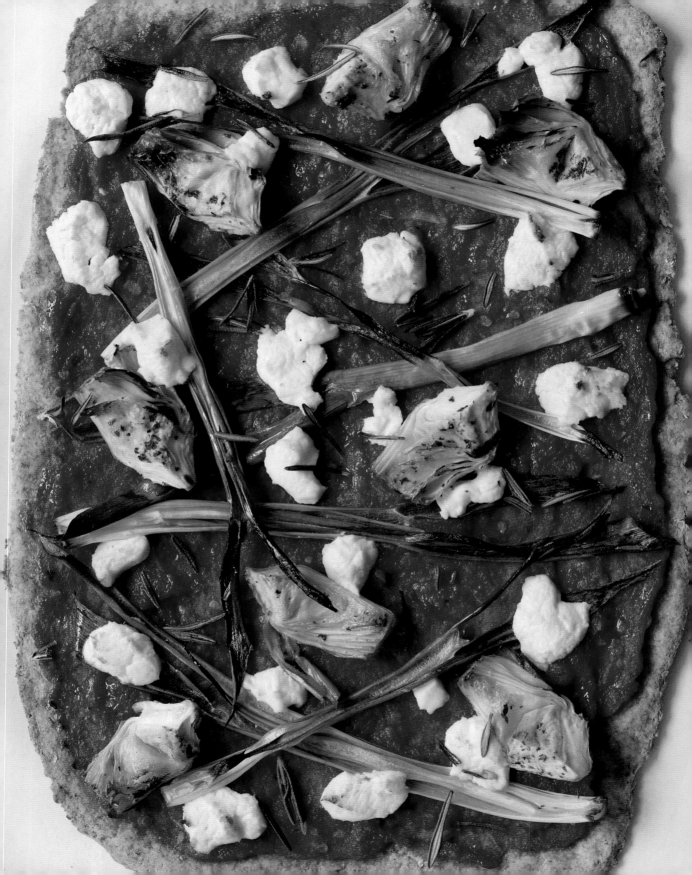

Spelt pizza with scallions, artichokes, and rosemary

This is my take on traditional family TV food, except this pizza will leave you with a spring in your step instead of a heavy, dull ache. You can change the toppings if you like but, if you are on a detox, artichoke is great for the liver and tomatoes are an antioxidant. The herbs also help with immunity and rosemary is said to improve memory. **MAKES 2 LARGE PIZZAS / SERVES 4**

1 Begin by making the sauce for the topping. Place the onion and garlic in the bowl of a food processor and blitz until finely pureed. Heat the oil in a frying pan and add the onion and garlic mix. Fry gently for five minutes, until cooked through and slightly golden. Meanwhile, blitz the tomatoes in a food processor until pureed. Add the tomatoes to the cooked onion mix, with the oregano and salt. Continue to cook the mixture until thickened; this should take about five minutes. Set aside to cool.

2 Preheat the oven to 475°F [220°C]. To make the dough, sift the flour into a mixing bowl and stir in the salt and baking powder. Make a well in the center and pour in the oil and up to ⅝ cup [150 ml] of warm filtered water to make a firm dough. Bring together with your hands, adding a little extra filtered water if necessary, and knead briefly.

3 Divide the dough into two and roll out on two lightly floured, nonstick baking sheets into large rectangles. Spoon over the sauce and spread it out over the base, then sprinkle the remaining toppings over the two pizzas.

4 Bake in the oven for eight to 10 minutes, until the base is burnished and the toppings are golden. Serve immediately.

FOR THE TOPPING

½ onion, cut into large chunks

1 garlic clove, peeled

1 tsp avocado oil

4 large tomatoes, peeled (see page 119), seeded, and coarsely chopped

½ tsp dried oregano

pinch of Himalayan or Celtic salt

4 artichoke hearts in oil, drained and sliced

8 scallions, sliced lengthwise

2 tsp coarsely chopped rosemary leaves

1¾ oz [50 g] goat cheese (optional), crumbled or grated

FOR THE DOUGH

2 cups [250 g] whole grain spelt flour, plus more to dust

pinch of Himalayan or Celtic salt

2 tsp baking powder

2 tsp coconut oil, melted

Beet and quinoa burger

Giving up meat? Hopefully the color and texture of this veggie burger will satisfy any carnivorous cravings. Your body gets the same high quantity of iron as it would from meat (from the beet), plus antioxidants (from the veg) and more easily absorbable protein (from the quinoa and eggs). You can add a fried egg on top if you really feel in need of a bigger protein punch. **SERVES 4**

1 Trim, peel, and coarsely grate the beets and the carrot. Put all the ingredients except the oil into a large bowl and mix thoroughly.

2 Shape the mixture into four patties and gently steam-fry them in the oil (see page 9) until crispy on both sides and heated through.

2 medium beets

1 large carrot

½ cup [110 g] cooked quinoa (see page 89) or aduki beans

1 onion, minced

2 eggs, lightly beaten

scant 1 cup [100 g] buckwheat flour

½ tsp fennel seeds

1 tsp coconut oil

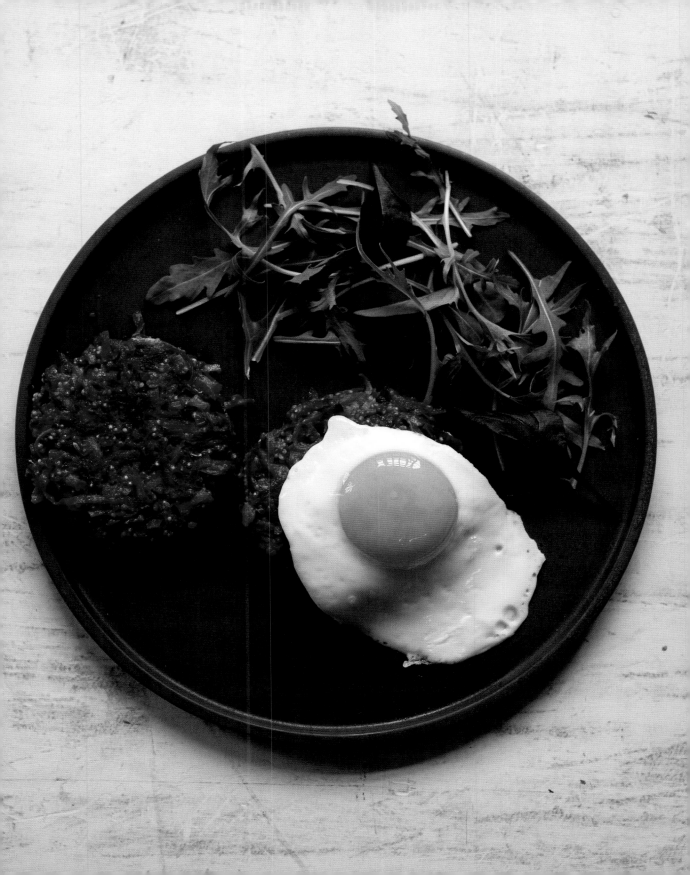

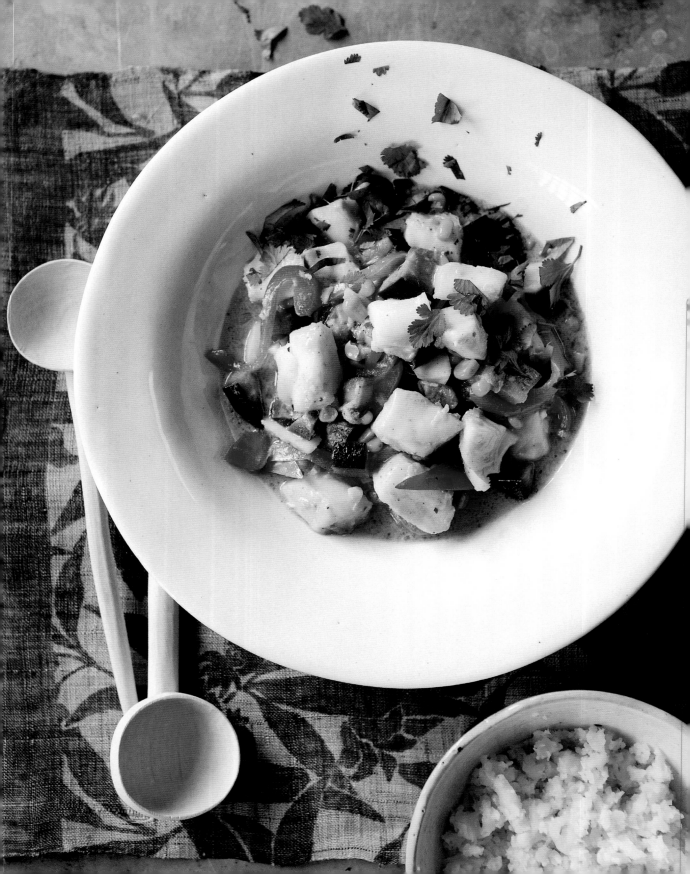

Thai fish curry

Lighter than Indian fish curry (see page 116), this is a nice dish for summer eating. It is very alkalizing and nutrient-dense (especially if you use my vegetable broth recipe, see page 79). The spices liven up the digestion, while coconut alkalizes to give a very "clean" taste. You can make the base of this the night before and let the flavors mellow a bit, then heat it through, place the fish on top, and steam it. **SERVES 2**

1 Fry the curry paste and lemon grass in the coconut milk until the mixture is thick and very aromatic. Add the eggplant, lime leaves, garlic, and ginger, cover, and simmer, but do not overcook. Add the bell peppers and corn and cook for a few minutes.

2 Add the broth a little at a time, keeping the thickness of the curry. Add the amino acids or salt. Simmer for a while, then place the fish on top, cover, and steam until cooked. Sprinkle with cilantro and serve.

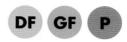

1 to 2 tsp green Thai curry paste, to taste (make your own or buy it)

1 lemon grass stalk, trimmed and thinly sliced

5 Tbsp [75 ml] organic coconut milk, ideally homemade (see page 46)

3½ oz [100 g] eggplant, chopped into cubes

3 kaffir lime leaves, shredded

2 garlic cloves, crushed

1-in [2.5-cm] piece of gingerroot, minced or grated

¼ red bell pepper, thinly sliced

¼ orange bell pepper, thinly sliced

3½ oz [100 g] corn, shaved from the cob

⅝ cup [150 ml] vegetable broth, ideally homemade (see page 79)

4 drops of liquid amino acids, or a pinch of Himalayan or Celtic salt

2 pieces of white fish (haddock, monkfish, red snapper, flounder), chopped into bite-size pieces, if you like

handful of chopped cilantro

Salmon and salsa "sandwiches" with quinoa

Salmon is a fabulous source of protein and omega-3 fatty acids. This light meal can be served up at a dinner party and anyone suffering from joint pain, a cold, or a bit of the blues will thank you as it is full of antioxidants and immune-boosting herbs, and it delivers a serotonin high. **SERVES 2**

1 For the salsa, put all the ingredients except the oil in a blender and pulse-blend. Add olive oil, little by little, until it is the consistency of pesto. Preheat the oven to 400°F [200°C].

2 Put the quinoa, broth, and saffron into a pan and bring to a boil. Simmer for about 10 minutes, just until the broth has almost evaporated, then turn the heat off and cover the pan. The quinoa will puff up and absorb the remaining liquid on its own. Let rest.

3 Blend the almonds and oats together to make a flour. Add the oat flour to the 4 teaspoons of salsa and mix into a paste.

4 Remove the skin from each piece of salmon and carefully cut the fillets horizontally so each is like a sandwich. Spread the salsa mix between the pieces of salmon, as if it were the sandwich filling, reassembling each fillet afterward. Place on a baking sheet and cook for 10 minutes.

5 Meanwhile, steam-fry the leek (see page 9) in a little filtered water and the coconut oil.

6 Mix the tomatoes into the warm quinoa; they will soften in the heat. Put some quinoa on each plate, place the salmon on top, and sprinkle the leeks over. Serve with Broiled zucchini salad with garlic and basil (see page 129).

FOR THE GREEN SALSA

3½ oz [100 g] spinach

3⅓ cups [100 g] Italian parsley

4¼ cups [100 g] basil

2 garlic cloves, peeled

¼ onion

1 chile, seeded

⅝ cup [150 ml] cider vinegar

juice of 1 lemon

olive oil

FOR THE SALMON AND QUINOA

¾ cup [150 g] quinoa

2 cups [500 ml] vegetable broth, ideally homemade (see page 79)

6 saffron strands

scant ¼ cup [20 g] almonds

¼ cup [20 g] oats

4 tsp Green salsa (see above)

2 x salmon fillets

1 leek, sliced

1 tsp coconut oil

2 tomatoes, chopped

Edamame rice bowls

Shelled edamame (soybeans) are a fabulous way of getting fat-free protein. They taste delicious and are filling and health-enhancing. You can steam them in their pods and eat them just with a pinch of salt but, if you want a meal, here is a good option. **SERVES 2**

1 Bring 1¼ cups [300 ml] of filtered water to a boil and stir in the rice. Cover, reduce the heat to medium-low, and simmer for 45 minutes, or until the water has almost evaporated. Turn the heat off, put a lid on the saucepan, and let rest.

2 Bring 1⅔ cups [400 ml] of filtered water to a boil, add the edamame beans, and cook for about two minutes, or until tender, then drain and set aside.

3 Chop the radishes. Scoop the seeds out of the pomegranate.

4 Combine the rice, edamame, radishes, pomegranate, goji berries, cilantro, olives, sea vegetables, and red pepper flakes in a large bowl.

5 Mix the olive oil and lime juice and gently fold into the rice.

FOR THE RICE BOWLS

scant ½ cup [80 g] whole grain or wild rice

7¾ oz [225 g] frozen edamame beans

4 radishes

½ pomegranate

¼ cup [30 g] goji berries

3 Tbsp chopped cilantro

10 pitted kalamata olives, halved

1 tsp mixed dried sea vegetables

¼ tsp red pepper flakes

FOR THE DRESSING

1 Tbsp olive oil

1 Tbsp lime juice

Split pea dhal

Alkalizing, anti-inflammatory, high in fiber, and cholesterol-reducing, this supereasy dish is also a good detoxer, as split peas are high in molybdenum, a mineral that metabolizes sulfites (preservatives) and alcohol. Plus it's filling. Eat as a main meal or a side with curry. **SERVES 4 SMALL OR 2 BIG APPETITES**

1 Pour the peas into a pitcher and note their volume. Tip into a colander and wash well. Put in a pan with five times their volume of filtered water. Bring to a boil, then simmer for 35 minutes or until tender. Drain and rinse thoroughly.

2 Sauté the garlic and onion in the coconut oil until translucent. Add the spices and salt and cook for two minutes, stirring. Add the cooked split peas and coat them in the spices, then pour in the coconut milk. Simmer gently for about 20 minutes, adding a little filtered water if the mixture becomes too thick.

1 cup [200 g] dried split peas

1 garlic clove, crushed

½ onion, minced

1 tsp coconut oil

1 tsp ground turmeric

½ tsp cayenne pepper

½ tsp red pepper flakes

¼ tsp Himalayan or Celtic salt

1⅔ cups [400 ml] organic coconut milk, ideally homemade (see page 46)

Zucchini spaghetti with tomato and pine nuts

Good for detox and weight loss, cholesterol-reducing, inflammation-busting, and antioxidant, this is youthing on a plate. It's pretty yummy too and, if you cut and cook the zucchini right, they'll eat just like al dente pasta. **SERVES 2**

1 Wash the zucchini thoroughly and, with a peeler or a mandolin—or a spiralizer, if you have one—slice into thin slices, or, if you like a thicker feel, cut lengthwise into small thick strips, like spaghetti.

2 Peel the tomatoes: make a small cross-shaped incision at the base of each, then dip in boiling water for 15 seconds or until the skin is beginning to come away from the flesh. Remove the tomatoes with a slotted spoon and plunge into ice-cold water. Carefully peel the skins away, then chop the tomatoes very finely.

3 Roast the pine nuts until lightly bronzed: place the pine nuts in a dry skillet over medium heat and cook, stirring, until they turn a shade darker and smell toasted. Tip out onto a plate to cool and stop the cooking.

4 Put 7 Tbsp [100 ml] of the broth in a pan with the tomatoes and ginger and simmer slowly for about five minutes, or until the broth has reduced. Add the rest of the broth and the zucchini. Simmer for another minute and a half or until the zucchini have wilted. Tear in the basil and mix together.

5 Take off the heat and sprinkle with the pine nuts.

2 zucchini
2 tomatoes
1/3 cup [50 g] pine nuts
5/8 cup [150 ml] vegetable broth, ideally homemade (see page 79)
3/4-oz [20 g] piece of gingerroot, minced
8 basil leaves

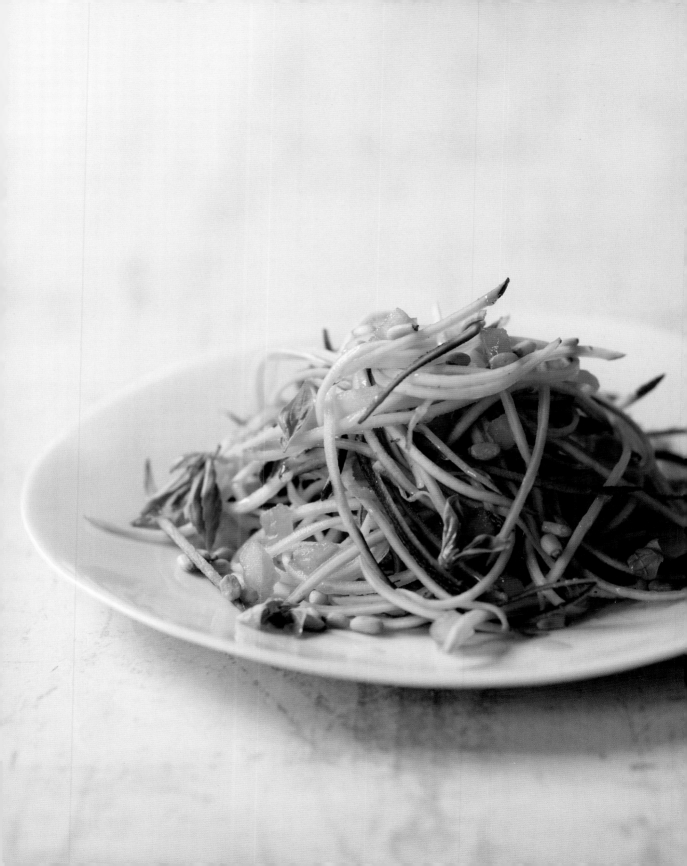

Indian fish curry

Indian food is an easy way to eat therapeutic, youthing spices in large quantities. What with the white fish and root veg, this is a protein- and omega-3-rich dish which tastes substantial and meaty. You can make the vegetable base of this curry the night before, then heat it through and place the fish on top to steam. This will also give a chance to let the spices mellow. **SERVES** 2

1 Pour about scant ¼ cup [50 ml] of the coconut milk into a hot pan and let it simmer for 90 seconds, to reduce and thicken. Add the ginger, curry powder, turmeric, horseradish, cardamom, garlic, curry leaves, star anise, and another ⅝ cup [150 ml] of the coconut milk.

2 Now add the eggplant, potato, and squash and let it simmer, adding small amounts of coconut milk to prevent it from getting too dry, until it has all been used up. Then start adding splashes of filtered water when needed—up to a maximum of 5 Tbsp [75 ml]—until it, too, is all used up. Cover and simmer for three to four minutes, then season with the salt or sea vegetables.

3 When the vegetables are cooked, place the fish and shrimp on top, replace the lid, and steam the fish for about two minutes. Gently stir in the mango. Serve, sprinkled with cilantro, with lime wedges on the side.

1¼ cups [300 ml] organic coconut milk, ideally homemade (see page 46)

⅓-oz [10-g] gingerroot, minced

3 tsp mild curry powder

2 tsp ground turmeric

1 tsp noncreamy horseradish (read the label!)

4 cardamom pods, crushed

1 garlic clove, crushed

3 curry leaves

2 star anise

3½ oz [100 g] eggplant, chopped

3½ oz [100 g] new potato, chopped

3½ oz [100 g] butternut squash, chopped

pinch of Himalayan or Celtic salt or mixed dried sea vegetables

2 fillets of firm white fish, cut into bite-size pieces

4 large shrimp

1¾ oz [50 g] green mango, or regular mango, finely chopped

handful of chopped cilantro, to serve

lime wedges, to serve

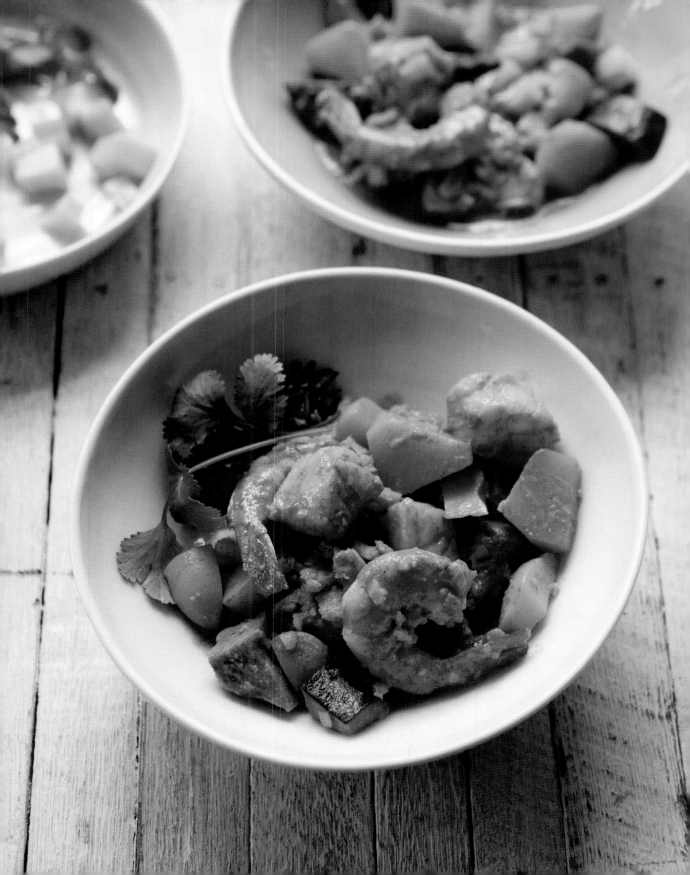

Cod Provençal

One of my dinner party favorites, this is supereasy to make but looks almost Cordon Bleu. **SERVES 4**

1 Preheat the oven to 350°F [180°C].

2 Heat the oil in a large ovenproof frying pan over medium-low heat. Add the onion, garlic, and oregano and fry gently for two or three minutes, until beginning to soften. Add the pepper and fry for another two or three minutes, until everything is soft and golden.

3 Add the cod fillets and fry for a minute on each side. Tip in the tomatoes and olives and bring to a simmer.

4 Transfer the pan to the oven and bake for 10 to 12 minutes, until the fish is opaque and cooked through. If you think it could do with a little more color, pop it under a hot broiler for a couple of minutes. Sprinkle with the lemon juice, season with the pepper, and sprinkle over the basil to serve.

2 tsp avocado or coconut oil

1 medium onion, chopped

2 garlic cloves, minced

2 tsp minced oregano leaves

1 red bell pepper, finely sliced

4 cod fillets

4 large tomatoes, seeded, chopped

6 pitted black olives, halved

juice of ½ lemon

¼ tsp freshly ground black pepper

handful of basil leaves, shredded

Steamed Asian fragrant fish with sesame broccoli

The aromatics here—ginger, onion, garlic, and chile—get your stomach ready for digestion. Served with Sesame broccoli (see page 129) this is an alkalizing, anti-inflammatory meal. **SERVES 4**

1 Preheat the oven to 350°F [180°C]. Lay out four large sheets of parchment paper and fold them in half vertically. Draw out a half heart shape on the top piece of paper (large enough to fit one fish fillet) and cut out. Unfurl the paper to make four hearts and place a fillet on one side of each heart. Sprinkle the remaining ingredients between the fillets.

2 Lay the top side of each heart over the fish and, starting at the pointed end, crimp the paper at the edges to envelop the fish. Repeat with the remaining packages and transfer them all to a baking sheet, spacing them out well.

3 Bake for 10 to 12 minutes, until the paper is golden and the packs have puffed up with steam. To serve, cut open each package to release the delicious aromas.

4 x 4¼-oz [120-g] white fish fillets, such as sea bass, haddock, or pollack

4 scallions, finely sliced

1-in [2.5-cm] piece of gingerroot, shredded

2 garlic cloves, finely sliced

2 to 4 Thai chiles (depending how hot you like it), finely sliced

2 tsp liquid amino acids

1 tsp coconut oil, melted

Sesame broccoli (see page 129), to serve

Zucchini spaghetti with squid

Squid is a light protein source that adds a delicious texture to a dish. Zucchini are high in fiber, vitamins, antioxidants, help reduce cholesterol ... and make zany spaghetti! Spiced with fragrant European herbs that are good for digestion and high in vitamin D, this is tasty, wholesome, and youthing. **SERVES 4**

2¼ lb [1 kg] squid, cleaned

2 large zucchini

scant ¼ cup [50 ml] vegetable broth, ideally homemade (see page 79)

2 tsp ground ginger

1 tsp coconut oil

½ tsp chopped mint leaves

½ tsp chopped basil leaves

½ tsp chopped parsley leaves

1 tsp lemon juice

1 Wash the squid, then cut off both ends of the tubes (set the tentacles aside). Cut down one side to open out the tubes, then scrape the inner surface clean with the blunt edge of a knife. Slice through to create two halves. Make crisscross score marks on the inside of the squid, being careful not to cut through. You can now either cut the squid into thin strips that will mix easily with the zucchini spaghetti, or cut each into four quarters, which will curl up when cooked and sit on the top.

2 Wash the zucchini thoroughly and with a peeler or a mandolin—or a spiralizer, if you have one—slice into thin slices, or, if you like a thicker feel, cut lengthwise into small thick strips, like spaghetti.

3 Simmer the zucchini in the broth and ginger; keep turning until the zucchini is limp.

4 Steam-fry the squid (see page 9) in the coconut oil until it has curled up and is a solid white color.

5 When the zucchini and squid are ready, mix them together and sprinkle with the herbs and lemon juice.

10
SIDE DISHES

'Age is something that does not matter, unless you are a cheese,'

LUIS BUÑUEL

Lima bean puree

I love lima beans and, unlike some other beans, they don't give you wind! They are a fabulous source of protein, high in fiber, and mineral-dense. If you make too much of this puree, add chickpeas to it and you have a youthing houmous!
MAKES ABOUT 9 OZ [250 G] SERVES 4

½ cup [100 g] dried lima beans

½ garlic clove, minced or crushed

2 Tbsp olive oil

juice of ½ lemon

Himalayan or Celtic salt

freshly ground black pepper

1 To cook the lima beans, soak overnight in cold filtered water. Rinse under filtered water. Pour them into a measuring cup and make a note of their volume.

2 Place in a large pan with double their volume of filtered water and bring to a boil. Boil rapidly for 10 minutes, then reduce the heat and simmer for 20 minutes, or until tender. Do not add salt. Drain, setting aside the cooking liquid.

3 To make the puree, place all the ingredients in a blender and pulse-blend, adding splashes of cooking liquid as you need them, until you have a puree with a consistency you like. Season with salt and black pepper to taste. This can take a lot of seasoning, but don't go too mad with the salt.

Cauliflower puree

High in fiber and with the ability to neutralize potential toxins, cauliflower is a must-have in any detox. This is a deliciously creamy way of eating it and is wonderful as a side dish with fish or chicken. **SERVES 4**

1 cauliflower

freshly ground black pepper

½ tsp freshly grated nutmeg

generous 1 cup [250 ml] almond milk

1 Break up the cauliflower with your fingers or a knife, place it in a steamer and steam for eight to 10 minutes, or until soft.

2 Place in a blender with black pepper, the nutmeg, and almond milk. Blend to a smooth puree.

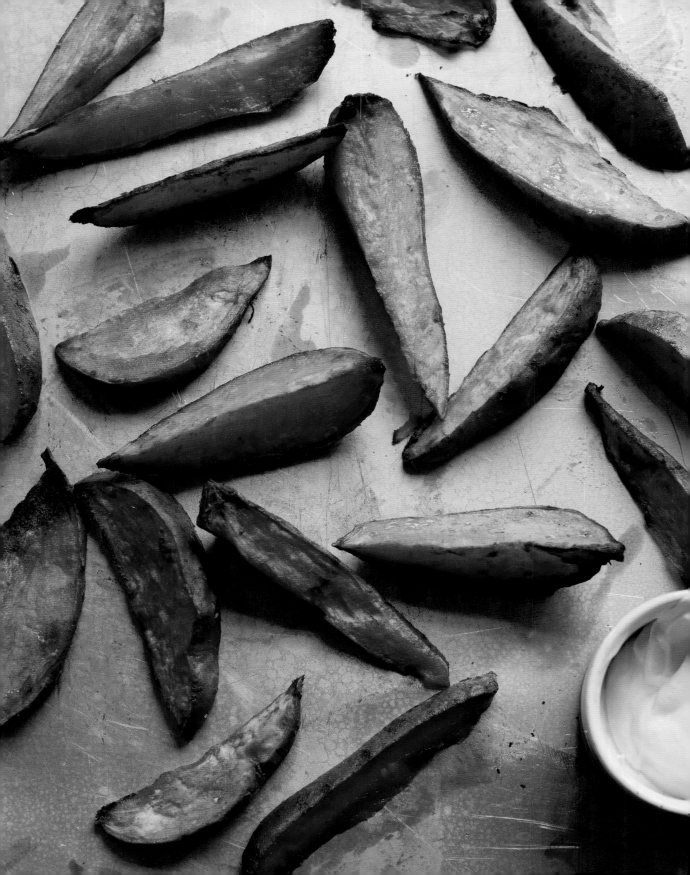

Sweet potato wedges

If you want something more exotic than regular French fries, sweet potatoes are the way to go. They taste deliciously vibrant, are rich in antioxidants, and will keep your gut in great shape. They're also thought to help your body produce sex hormones (via the carotenes they contain) and boost the thyroid, which is your metabolic marker and energizer. This is as youthful as it gets! **SERVES 4**

1 Preheat the oven to 400°F [200°C]. Begin by tossing the sweet potato wedges in the paprika and oil.

2 Tumble into a shallow roasting pan and bake for 20 to 35 minutes, turning occasionally, until crisp outside but tender within.

2 medium sweet potatoes, cut into wedges

½ tsp paprika

1 tsp avocado or coconut oil, melted, to taste

Roast cauliflower "rice"

Another great way of using cauliflower. Its detox effects will keep your liver healthy, your skin clear, and your gut running optimally. Keep eating it in any way you can. **SERVES 4**

1 Preheat the oven to 400°F [200°C].

2 Whiz the cauliflower in a food processor until it resembles grains of rice. Toss in the oil and transfer to a baking sheet.

3 Roast for 15 to 20 minutes, until golden and tender.

1 cauliflower, cut into florets

½ tsp coconut oil, melted

Eggplant-coconut rolls

I went to Greece when I was 17 and fell in love … with eggplant! Baked, stuffed, dried, in moussaka, you name it, I ate it. This dish is light but filling and mixes my favorite ingredient with nori seaweed, which is therapeutically powerful. **SERVES 2**

1 Blitz the coconut in a food processor until ground.

2 Slice the eggplant into long thin strips, about ¼ in [5 mm] thick, using a mandolin or a very sharp knife.

3 Using a vegetable peeler, slice the zucchini lengthwise into ribbons.

4 Mix the seeds, pine nuts, and coconut together with the olive oil, lime juice, and herbs.

5 Cook the eggplant and zucchini by dry-frying them on a hot griddle or grill pan. Don't overcook them; they should remain firm.

6 Put a zucchini slice on a board, place an eggplant slice on top, then put some coconut mixture in the middle and roll. Cut a strip from a nori sheet, wet it, and wrap it around the roll to hold it together.

7 Repeat to make more rolls, then serve immediately.

5¼ oz [150 g] coconut flesh, chopped

1 medium eggplant

1 medium zucchini

1 Tbsp sesame seeds

1 Tbsp black poppy seeds

1 Tbsp pine nuts

2 tsp olive oil

1 tsp lime juice

1 tsp mixed chopped parsley and basil leaves

1 sheet of nori seaweed

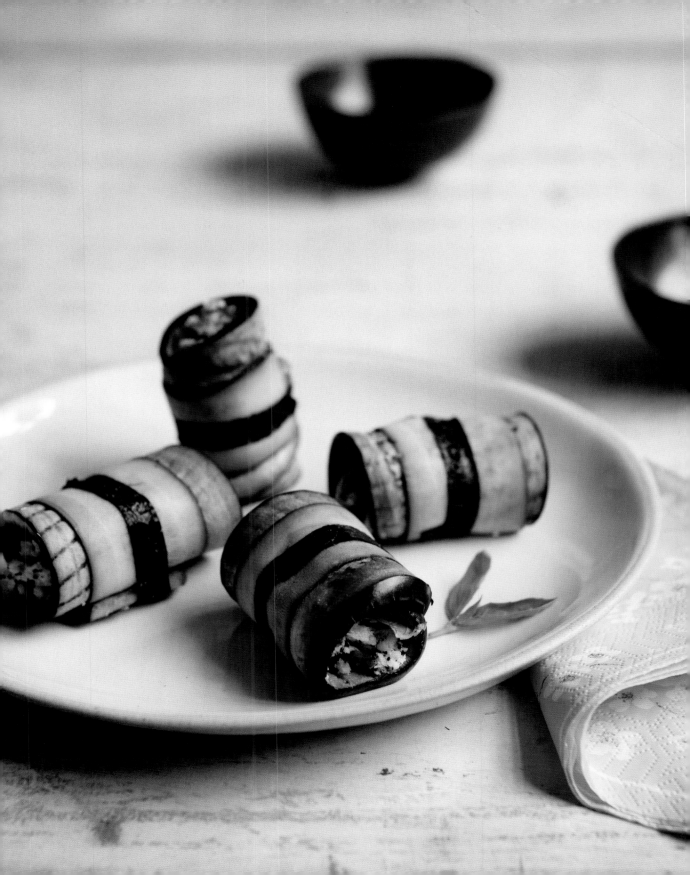

Special guacamole

Avocado is pretty much a mainstay of my diet. I eat it as often as I can. I love the taste; while its creamy texture lends itself well to smoothies and salads and is simply delicious in this traditional guacamole. Avocado contains a rich supply of vitamins, twice as much potassium as a banana, and is rich in omega fatty acids to keep skin youthful and hair luscious. **SERVES 4 TO 6**

1 Gently toast the pumpkin seeds in a dry frying pan.

2 Blend everything in a food processor for 30 to 45 seconds; the mixture should retain a slightly chunky texture.

½ cup [66 g] pumpkin seeds

2 ripe avocados, pitted and peeled

2 cups [230 g] cooked peas

1 garlic clove

large handful of mint leaves

finely grated zest and juice of 1 unwaxed lemon

1 Tbsp extra virgin olive oil

Himalayan or Celtic salt

freshly ground black pepper

Beet salsa

Beet is a powerful detoxer that revitalizes your whole system. It's packed with iron, calcium, magnesium, and other important minerals, bursting with wonderful antioxidants, vitamins, and anti-inflammatories and full of fiber for great gut youthing. Made like this, you can eat a good amount of it on Mixed seed crackers (see page 53), with fish or raw vegetables. **SERVES 4**

1 Put the beets in a pan, cover with filtered water, and bring to a boil. Simmer for about 20 minutes, then drain and cool. Peel (you might want to protect your hands as beet stains), then cut into ⅜-in [1-cm] dice.

2 Mix with the scallions and lemon juice.

2 beets

2 scallions, minced

juice of 1 lemon

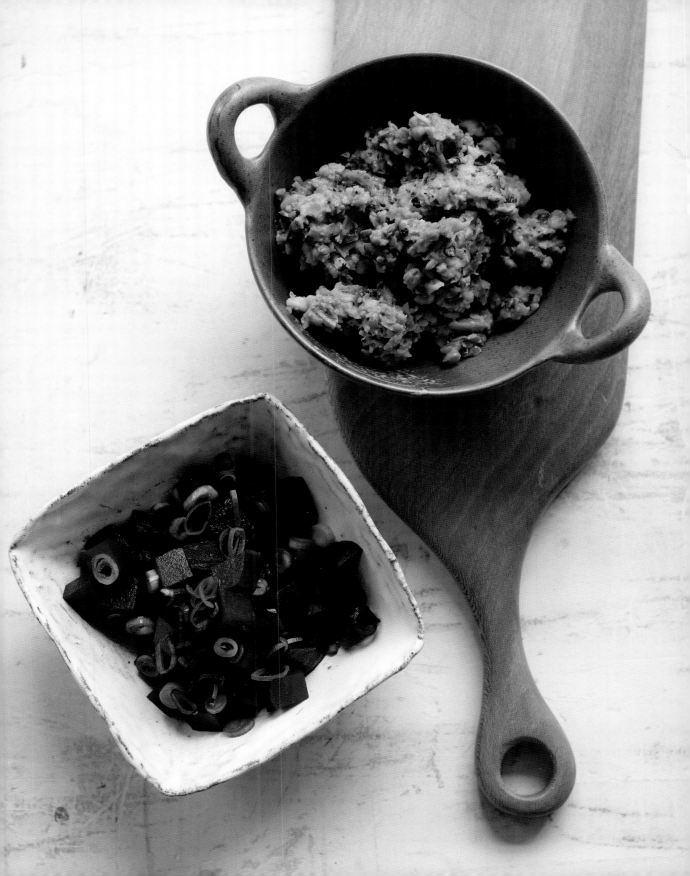

Sweet potato and fenugreek curry

Fenugreek has a bittersweet maple syrupy flavor and is often used in Indian and Middle Eastern cooking. It can reduce "bad" cholesterol and blood sugar levels, so helps to protect against diabetes. This curry is deliciously hot (thanks to the nigella and red pepper flakes) as a side dish, but just add some broccoli, cauliflower, or other fresh veg if you want to stretch it into a main to serve more people. **SERVES 4 TO 6 (DEPENDING IF IT'S A SIDE OR A MAIN)**

1 Peel the sweet potato and chop into 2-in [5-cm] squares. Peel and slice the onions quite finely.

2 Heat a pan (woks are good) and melt the coconut oil. Add the nigella seeds, wait until they crackle, then add the onions. Stir a few times, then add scant ¼ cup [50 ml] of filtered water. The onions should steam-fry (see page 9) for about three minutes, or until translucent.

3 Add the turmeric, fenugreek, and red pepper flakes, stir, and wait for a minute. Add the sweet potatoes and 1½ cups [350 ml] more filtered water. Keep an eye on the mixture as it simmers; the water will reduce, but the curry should still be liquid at this stage. As the sweet potatoes begin to soften, add the raisins for a sweeter taste (if you want). At this point you can also add any greens you want, such as broccoli florets or chopped zucchini, to make it more of a main course. Cook until all the vegetables are just tender, then serve.

2 sweet potatoes

2 onions

1 tsp coconut oil

1 tsp nigella seeds

1 tsp ground turmeric

3 tsp fenugreek leaves

½ tsp red pepper flakes (depending on how spicy you want it)

1½ Tbsp raisins (optional)

Broiled zucchini salad with garlic and basil

This is a lovely way to eat zucchini and get vitamins A and C, knowing full well you're also helping to reduce cholesterol and inflammation in the body. Yummy! **SERVES 4**

4 zucchini

4 garlic cloves

basil leaves

1 Wash the zucchini and slice at an angle about ⅜ in [1 cm] thick. Slice the garlic thinly at an angle.

2 Heat a cast-iron griddle pan or grill pan. Put the zucchini slices on it until they start to brown, then turn with a pair of tongs and repeat. At the last minute throw on the garlic slices until they also brown slightly.

3 Take the zucchini out of the pan and put into a bowl with the garlic and basil to serve.

Sesame broccoli

To stay youthful, your immune system needs to be strong, which is where broccoli comes in. It's also a mood food, rich in folic acid and other B-vitamins for your nervous system, and containing tryptophan which helps your body to produce the feel-good hormone serotonin. Sesame seeds can be allergenic, so leave them out if you are concerned; you could add 1 oz [30 g] of baked whole chestnuts instead. **SERVES 4**

1 tsp coconut oil

7¾-oz [220 g] pack of Tenderstem broccoli

1 Tbsp sesame seeds

1 tsp liquid amino acids

¼ tsp red pepper flakes, to serve

1 Heat the coconut oil in a large frying pan over medium heat and add the broccoli. Pour in 1 Tbsp of filtered water and steam-fry for two or three minutes (see page 9), until almost tender.

2 Add the sesame seeds and fry for another minute to toast. Serve sprinkled with the liquid amino acids and red pepper flakes.

"Cheesy" stuffed tomatoes

Tomatoes are such a lovely versatile vegetable. They contain lycopene which makes our skin less sensitive to UV light damage and so prevents lines and wrinkles. Plus they have vitamin K, calcium, and chromium to help regulate blood sugar levels … and I have not even got to the antioxidant value yet! This is a fabulously delicious way to eat them. **MAKES 4**

4 firm vine tomatoes

2 shallots

2 garlic cloves

1 tsp avocado oil, plus more to drizzle

2 Tbsp Creamy "cheese" (see page 81)

leaves from a small bunch of basil, chopped

1 Tbsp Walnut "Parmesan" (see page 81)

1 Preheat the oven to 350°F [180°C].

2 Wash the tomatoes, stand them on their bases, and slice off a "lid." Slice a tiny bit off the bases as well, if necessary, so they sit straight. Scoop out the seeds and flesh with a dessertspoon (set them aside in a bowl), being careful to make no holes as you don't want your stuffing to melt out.

3 Mince the shallots and garlic and steam-fry with the avocado oil (see page 9). Add the tomato insides and the "cheese" and mix well together, then add the basil. Stuff all the mixture back into the tomatoes and sprinkle with the walnut "Parmesan." Drizzle with a little avocado oil.

4 Bake in the oven for 25 minutes, or until the tomatoes are soft and cooked through and the topping is golden.

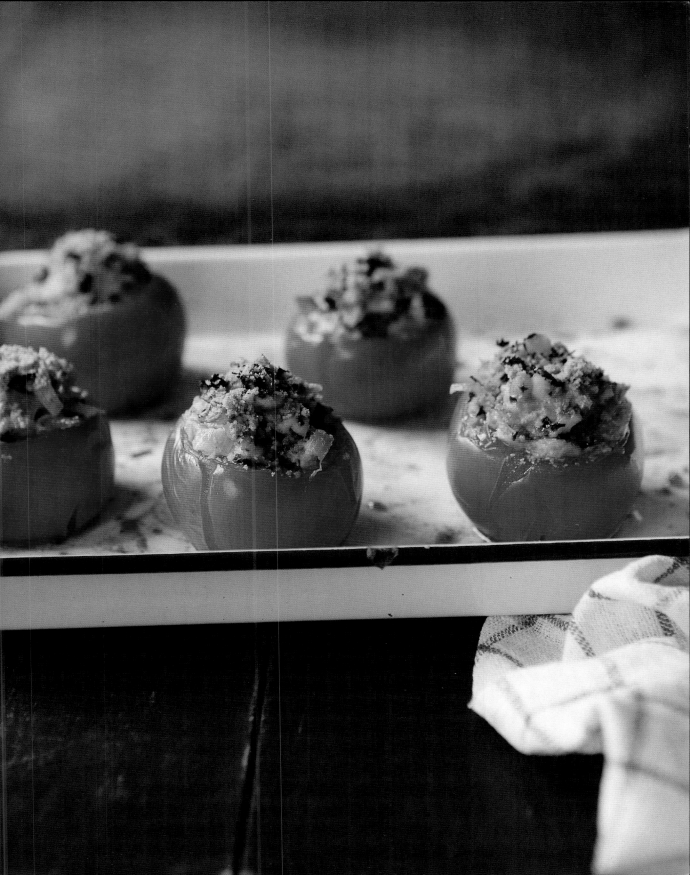

11
DESSERTS

'It's not what you look at that matters, it's what you see.'

HENRY DAVID THOREAU

It's hard to give up the traditional way of cooking desserts and sweet treats, but once you have mastered the basic CYY techniques you will find it supereasy and just as satisfying (if not more so) to make desserts that are youthing as well as delicious.

The only rule is that *sweet is sweet*, whether organic, plant-based, and natural (agave nectar, maple syrup, stevia, dates, and so on) or refined (white, brown, or powdered sugar).

If you want noticeable youthing results—clear, glowing skin, glossy hair and nails, a leaner body, and a more energized and positive approach—don't overeat any sugar. Think of sweet stuff as an occasional treat, not a must-have ending to every meal …

Cinnamon poached pears

Pears are very easy on the gut, as they're high in cholesterol-reducing pectin and fiber. The cinnamon in this recipe can help reduce blood sugar and lipid levels, making it a tasty treat for anyone who wants to look after their glucose levels. **MAKES 1**

1 Conference or Bosc pear, peeled and cored, stalk left on

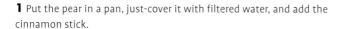

1 cinnamon stick

1 Put the pear in a pan, just-cover it with filtered water, and add the cinnamon stick.

2 Bring to a boil, then simmer for about 10 minutes, or until the pear is soft.

3 Remove the pear with a slotted spoon and reduce the remaining liquid in the pan by one-third until it begins to become syrupy (because of the pectin in the pear juice). Serve the pear with its syrupy spiced juice.

Raw vegan chocolate cheesecake

The best treat for anyone who's gluten- or dairy-free, raw, or vegan. It's simply delicious and rich in nuts, vanilla, and cinnamon … and so mood-enhancing and nutritious, too. But remember that sweet is sweet, so don't eat the whole thing and expect to feel youthful! Small slices work best. **SERVES 8**

1 For the filling, soak the cashews for two hours, then drain.

2 Meanwhile, for the crust, blend the nuts and dates in a food processor, add the cinnamon and coconut oil, and blend until well combined. Line the bottom of an 8-in [20-cm] springform cake pan with wax paper. Press the crust down evenly inside the pan so it is well compacted, then place in the freezer for 30 minutes to firm up.

3 Return to the filling: chop the zucchini into four pieces. Blend the drained cashews until smooth, then add the zucchini, cacao, maple syrup, vanilla, and salt. Finally, mix in the melted coconut oil. Blend until smooth, then spread over the top of the crust. Return to the freezer and let set.

4 Take the cheesecake from the freezer 30 minutes before serving. Slice the strawberries, sprinkle them with the pepper to bring out the flavor, then arrange them on top of the cheesecake, and sprinkle over the cacao nibs.

FOR THE FILLING

1¾ cups [260 g] raw cashews

1 small zucchini, peeled

¼ cup [25 g] raw cacao powder

¼ cup [85 g] maple syrup (optional)

1 Tbsp vanilla powder, or seeds of 1½ vanilla beans

¼ tsp Himalayan or Celtic salt

scant ¼ cup [43 g] coconut oil, melted

FOR THE CRUST

⅔ cup [100 g] almonds

⅔ cup [100 g] hazelnuts

3 oz [90 g] Medjool dates, pitted

½ tsp ground cinnamon (optional)

1½ Tbsp coconut oil

TO DECORATE

¾ cup [100 g] strawberries

pinch of black pepper

1 Tbsp cacao nibs

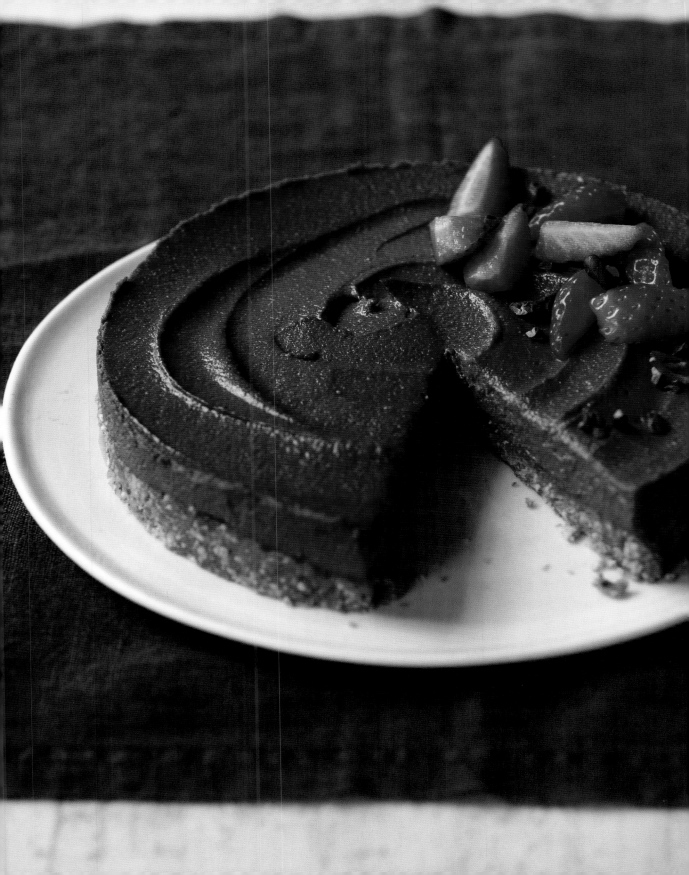

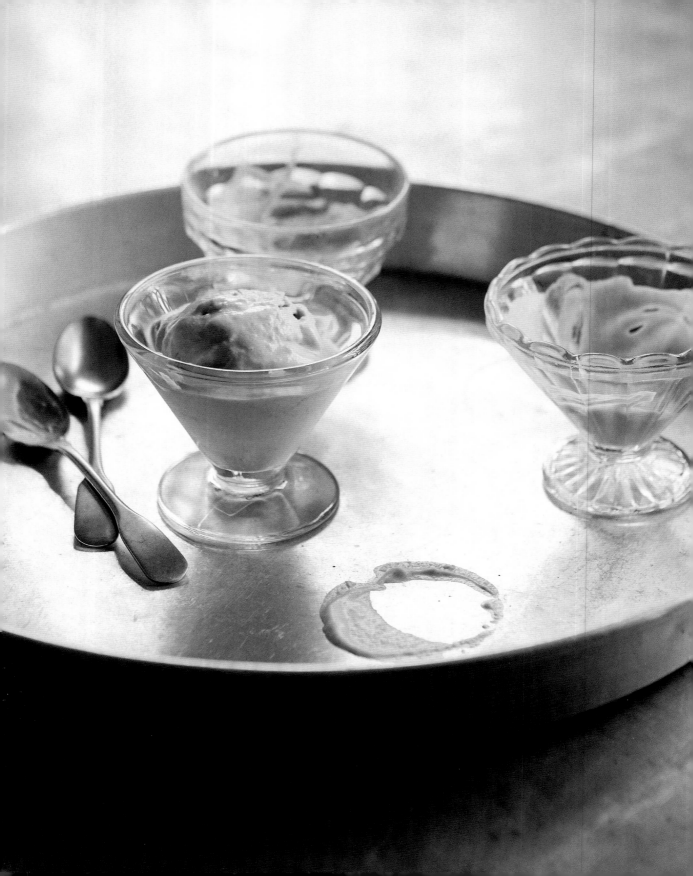

Almond, coconut, and vanilla ice cream

An extremely tasty nondairy ice cream that contains all-round great youthers: Dates are highly alkalizing and antioxidant, while vanilla gives you a bit of mood-lifting magic. Try it on family and friends and see … **SERVES 4 TO 6**

1 Put all the ingredients except the whole almonds in a blender and blitz until smooth. Preheat the oven to 325°F [160°C] and toast the almonds for five to 10 minutes. Coarsely chop them, then stir into the mixture.

2 Freeze in a shallow, freezerproof tray.

3 Before serving, break the frozen mass up and briefly whiz the frozen pieces in the blender, then scoop out and serve with berries or other fruit.

⅞ cup [200 ml] organic coconut milk, ideally homemade (see page 46)

1⅓ cups [120 g] ground almonds

10 dates, pitted

½ vanilla bean, seeds scraped out, or a few drops of vanilla extract

scant ½ cup [60 g] whole almonds

Pineapple and lemon sorbet

Pure fruit with nothing added. It's anti-inflammatory, good for digestion (both courtesy of the pineapple), and highly antioxidant, too. This sorbet is best eaten by itself, as the anti-inflammatory effects of bromelain (the enzyme in the pineapple) work better on an empty stomach. **SERVES 4 TO 6**

1 medium, ripe pineapple

juice of 1 lemon

1 Peel the pineapple by cutting the skin off vertically. Remove any "eyes" with the tip of the knife. Cut the fruit into rough chunks, discarding the woody core.

2 Place the pineapple in a large freezerproof dish and sprinkle over the lemon juice. Freeze for at least 12 hours.

3 Place the frozen pineapple in a food processor and blend until smooth, thick, and of a sorbet consistency. The sorbet can either be served straightaway or frozen until needed. If freezing, remove from the freezer 10 to 15 minutes before serving, to soften up.

Blackberry pastilles

I like to invent new ways of doing things, and using agar flakes seemed a perfect way to condense deliciously therapeutic blackberries into a tasty morsel. The deep blue color gives away the intensity of the youthing bioflavonoids and antioxidants served up in these fab desserts. **SERVES 8**

1¾ cups [250 g] blackberries (about 1 large carton), plus more to serve

3 apples

agar flakes (for amount, see recipe method)

Almond, coconut, and vanilla ice cream, to serve (see page 137)

1 Blend the blackberries until they are a puree. They have very small seeds so, if you don't like this rough taste, you need to blend them for a while and then strain the puree to make the mixture smooth. You should have about ⅞ cup [200 ml] of liquid by the time you have finished.

2 Put the apples into a juicer (if you don't have a juicer than use 2 Tbsp [35 ml] of organic cold-pressed juice instead); you should get about 2 Tbsp [35 ml] of fresh-extracted juice as well. Put the apple juice into a pan over medium heat and simmer until it reduces by half. Add the blended blackberries. Measure the volume of the liquid in the pan in a measuring cup and keep a note of it, then return it to the pan.

3 Sprinkle in 1 Tbsp of agar flakes per ⅞ cup [200 ml] of liquid and let simmer, without stirring. After it has simmered for one minute, stir occasionally until the flakes have disappeared.

4 Take off the heat and pour into an ice-cube tray. Let cool in the refrireratot. When the dessert has set, serve the cubes with Almond, coconut, and vanilla ice cream (see page 137) and fresh blackberries, or even just on their own. Or stick popsicle sticks in the cubes before freezing and eating as an ice pop.

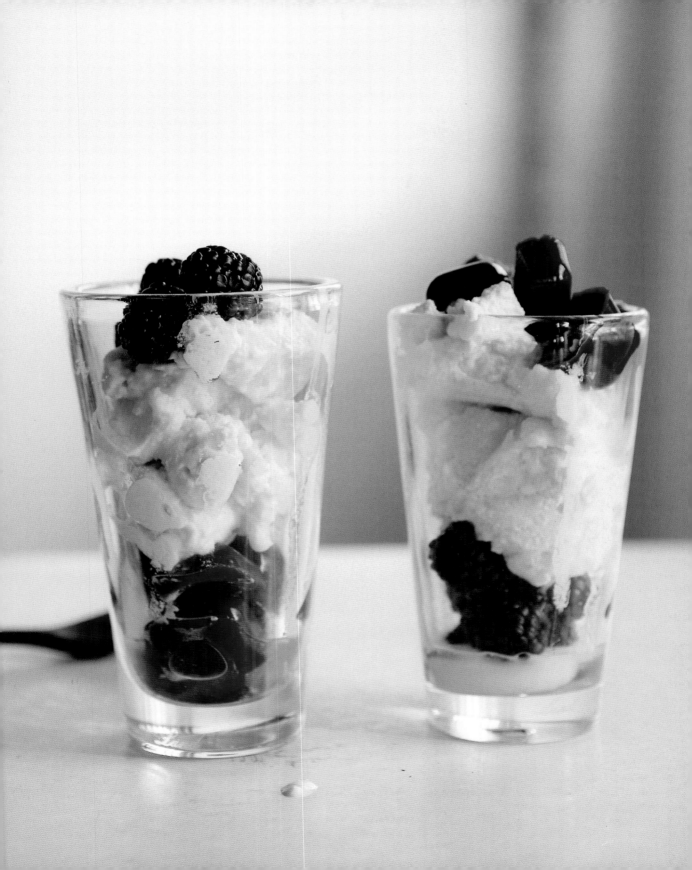

Citrus drizzle cake

A fruity cake with a tangy citrus zip that's much less sweet than a full-on lemon drizzle cake. It has good CYY benefits too: apricots contain lycopene and lutein (both antiaging carotenes), while coconut oil is a top youthing choice for both its waist-slimming and cholesterol-reducing properties. **ENOUGH FOR 12 SLICES**

1 Preheat the oven to 375°F [190°C]. Oil an 8-by-4-in [20-by-10-cm] loaf pan with a little coconut oil and line with parchment paper.

2 Place the lemon and orange zests and juices, maple syrup, apricots, and coconut oil in the bowl of a food processor and blitz until fairly smooth. Add the eggs and combine again. Pour the batter into a large bowl and fold in the ground almonds and baking powder.

3 Pour into the prepared pan and bake for 40 to 50 minutes, until golden brown and a skewer inserted into the center comes out clean. Let the cake cool for 10 minutes before turning out of the pan onto a wire rack.

4 Using a toothpick, pierce the warm cake liberally all over. Mix together the maple syrup and lemon juice in a small bowl. Pour the drizzle evenly over the top of the cake and serve while still warm.

DF **GF**

FOR THE CAKE

4 Tbsp coconut oil, melted, plus more for the pan

finely grated zest and juice of 1 unwaxed lemon

finely grated zest and juice of 1 medium orange

¼ cup [100 g] maple syrup (optional)

scant ½ cup [75 g] dried unsulfured apricots

4 large eggs, lightly beaten

3⅓ cups [300 g] ground almonds

1 tsp gluten-free baking powder, sifted

FOR THE DRIZZLE

1 Tbsp maple syrup (optional)

juice of ½ lemon

Macaroons

These make a nutritious showstopper dish sandwiched with coconut-cashew cream and served alongside Cinnamon poached pears (see page 133). Or simply eat them alone or with a dollop of ice cream. **MAKES 6 TO 8**

1 Preheat the oven to 350°F [180°C].

2 To make the macaroons, bring a small pan of water to a boil. Tip in the apricots and boil for one minute, then drain into a strainer. Finely chop the apricots and mix with the almonds until thoroughly combined. Add the maple syrup.

3 In a clean nonreactive bowl, whisk the egg whites to form soft peaks. Carefully fold the whites into the almond mixture with a metal spoon, using figure-eight movements.

4 Line a baking sheet with wax paper. Using a cookie cutter as a guide, drop the macaroon mixture into the cutter to make a small cookie. Repeat to use up all the macaroon mixture.

5 Bake for about 20 minutes, then take out of the oven and transfer the macaroons carefully to a wire rack to cool.

6 To make the coconut-cashew cream, place all the ingredients in a blender and blitz until smooth and creamy.

7 Take two of the macaroon rounds and sandwich together with the coconut-cashew cream. (You may have some cashew cream left over, so keep it for another day.)

FOR THE MACAROONS

¼ cup [50 g] dried unsulfured apricots

½ cup [50 g] ground almonds, or almond grounds from making almond milk

1 tsp maple syrup (optional)

2 egg whites

FOR THE COCONUT-CASHEW CREAM

7 Tbsp [100 ml] organic coconut milk, ideally homemade (see page 46)

scant 1 cup [130 g] raw cashews

2 dates, pitted

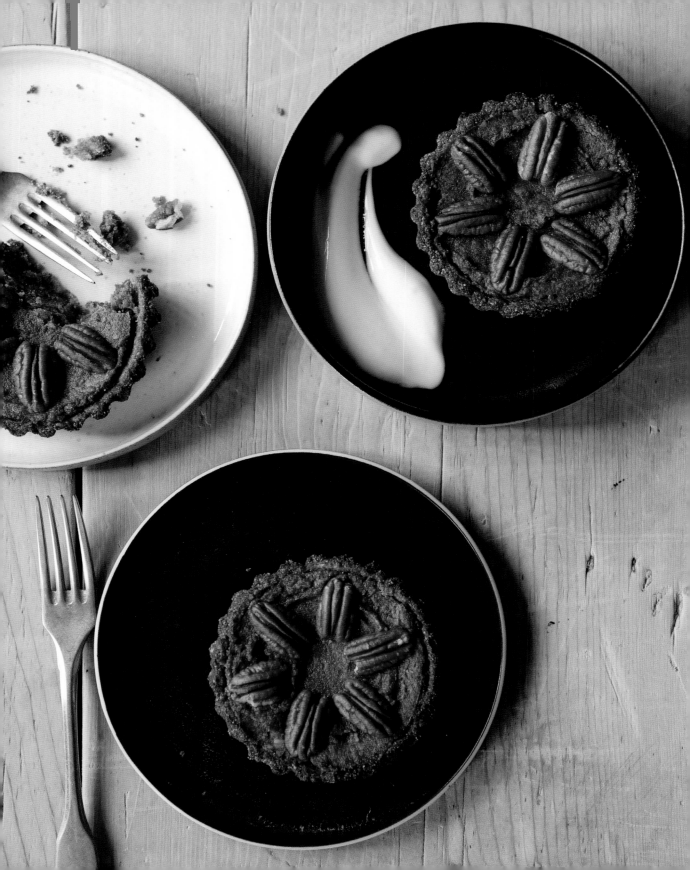

Pecan pies

When I was in America I loved the pecan pies people made at Thanksgiving. I never thought I'd be able to replicate a youthing version, but I have to say this is so close … and simply delicious. Pecans are very high in oleic acid which reduces cholesterol, full of phytochemicals which contribute to antioxidant activity, and are an excellent source of minerals, vitamin E, and several important B-complex vitamins. **MAKES 4 INDIVIDUAL PIES**

1 Begin by making the crust. Place the ground almonds, oats, cinnamon, dates, and oil in a food processor and blitz for about 30 seconds until you have a rough, doughy texture. Divide the "dough" into four and press each piece into a 4-in [10-cm] fluted tart shell. Chill in the refrigerator for at least 30 minutes to firm up.

2 Soak the dates for the filling in hot water for 15 minutes. Preheat the oven to 350°F [180°C].

3 To make the filling, place the drained dates, 1½ cups (220 g) of the pecans, and the remaining ingredients in a food processor and blitz until glossy and smooth. Spoon the filling into the four prepared shells and smooth the tops. Place a few of the reserved pecans on each pie.

4 Bake for 15 to 20 minutes, until the filling is set. Let cool in the pans for a few minutes before carefully turning out and serving. Delicious with vegan ice cream or yogurt.

FOR THE CRUST

2¼ cups [200 g] ground almonds

½ cup [50 g] rolled oats

¼ tsp ground cinnamon

5 Medjool dates, pitted

2 Tbsp coconut oil

FOR THE FILLING

12 Medjool dates, pitted

1⅔ cups [250 g] pecans

5 Tbsp almond milk

1 tsp ground cinnamon

1 tsp vanilla bean paste or vanilla extract

pinch of nutmeg

1 Tbsp coconut oil

½ tsp Himalayan or Celtic salt

Chocolate fix

Apple and walnut is a wonderful combination that becomes even more fabulous when chocolate is added; make it 85 percent cocoa solids for an extra youthing kick. **MAKES 12**

1 Line an 8-in [20-cm] square cake pan with parchment paper.

2 Put the apples in a pan with scant ¼ cup [50 ml] of filtered water and simmer for 10 minutes, or until the apple becomes a puree. Let cool. Preheat the oven to 350°F [180°C].

3 Place the chocolate in a heatproof bowl over a pan of very gently simmering water (the bowl should not touch the water) and let melt. Remove the bowl from the heat and set aside.

4 Tip the dates, stewed apple, eggs, and maple syrup into a food processor and blend until smooth. Scoop the mixture into a large bowl and fold in the flour, baking powder, and walnuts, followed by the slightly cooled chocolate. Spoon the mixture into the prepared pan and smooth over using a spatula.

5 Bake for 10 to 15 minutes, until spongy at the edges and still slightly sticky in the center. Let cool before either keeping as a cake, or cutting into squares like a brownie.

GF

4¼ oz (125 g/1½ to 2) eating apples, peeled, cored, and coarsely chopped

3½ oz [100 g] semisweet chocolate (ideally 85% cocoa solids), chopped small

20 dates, pitted

2 large eggs, lightly beaten

4 Tbsp maple syrup (optional)

½ cup [75 g] rice flour

½ tsp gluten-free baking powder

¼ cup [25 g] walnuts, coarsely chopped

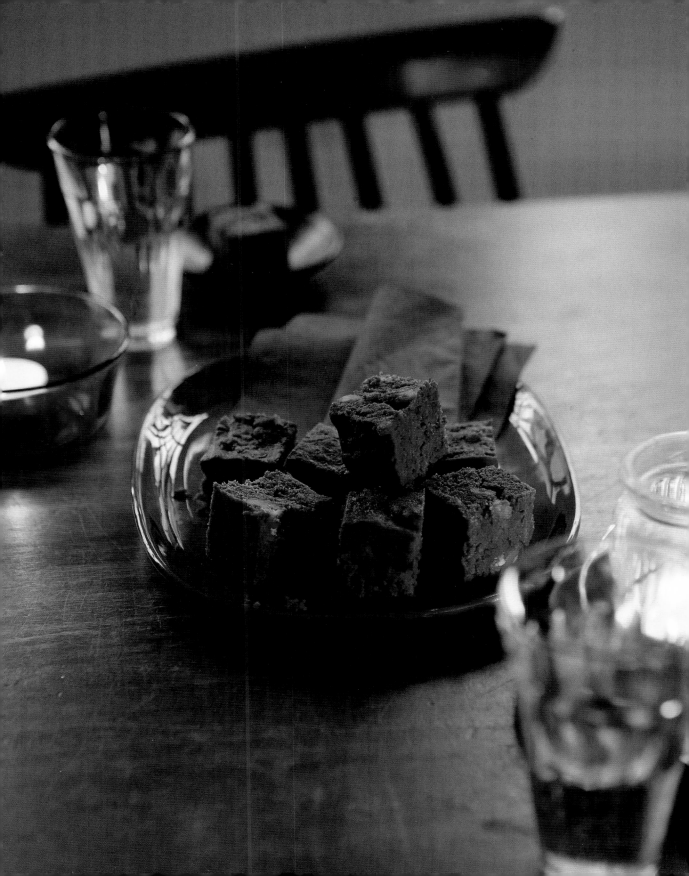

Biscotti

Whenever I get biscotti with my coffee or tea in an Italian restaurant, I pick out the almonds but have to leave the rest. It got me thinking that there must be a superdelicious way of making biscotti without gluten and refined sugar … well, bingo!
MAKES UP TO 12

3⅓ cups [300 g] ground almonds

2 Tbsp arrowroot

½ tsp baking soda

finely grated zest of 1 orange

4 Tbsp maple syrup (optional)
or Sweet apricot paste
(see page 71)

⅓ cup [50 g] pistachios

½ cup [50 g] cranberries

½ Tbsp coconut oil, melted

1 Preheat the oven to 400°F [200°C].

2 Pour the ground almonds, arrowroot, baking soda, and orange zest into a food processor and pulse briefly to combine. Now, with the motor running, gradually add the maple syrup or apricot paste to make a sticky dough.

3 Turn the dough out onto a counter and knead in the pistachios and cranberries. Shape the dough into a flattish log shape and place on a nonstick baking sheet. Bake for 15 minutes, then remove from the oven and let cool on a wire rack for 45 minutes.

4 Preheat the oven to 350°F [180°C]. Slice the biscotti log into ⅜ to ¾-in [1 to 2-cm] thick pieces and return to the baking sheet, cut sides up. Brush a little oil over each cookie and bake, turning once, for 20 to 25 minutes, until crisp and golden. Transfer carefully to a wire rack to cool. Store in an airtight container.

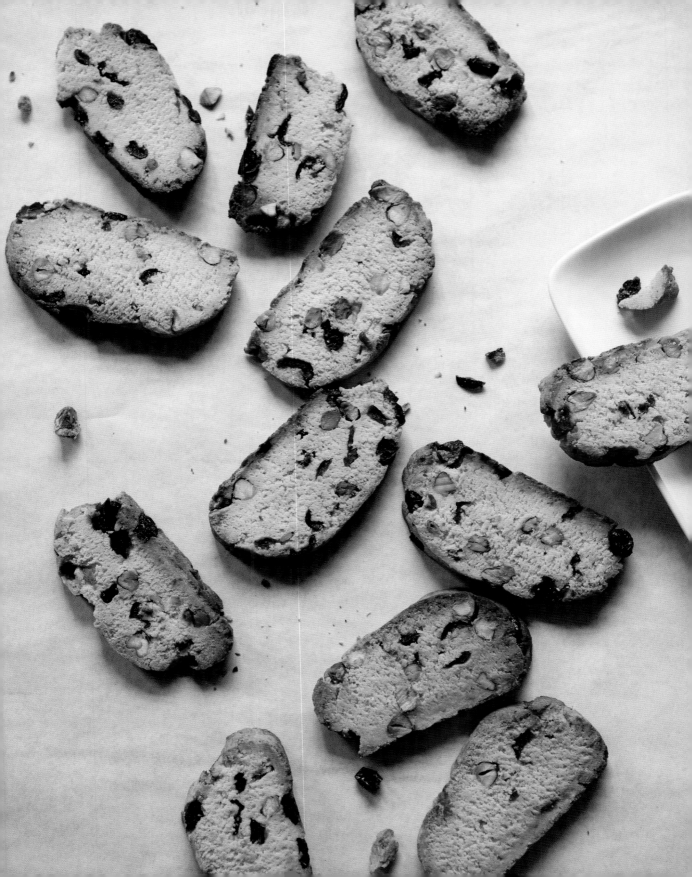

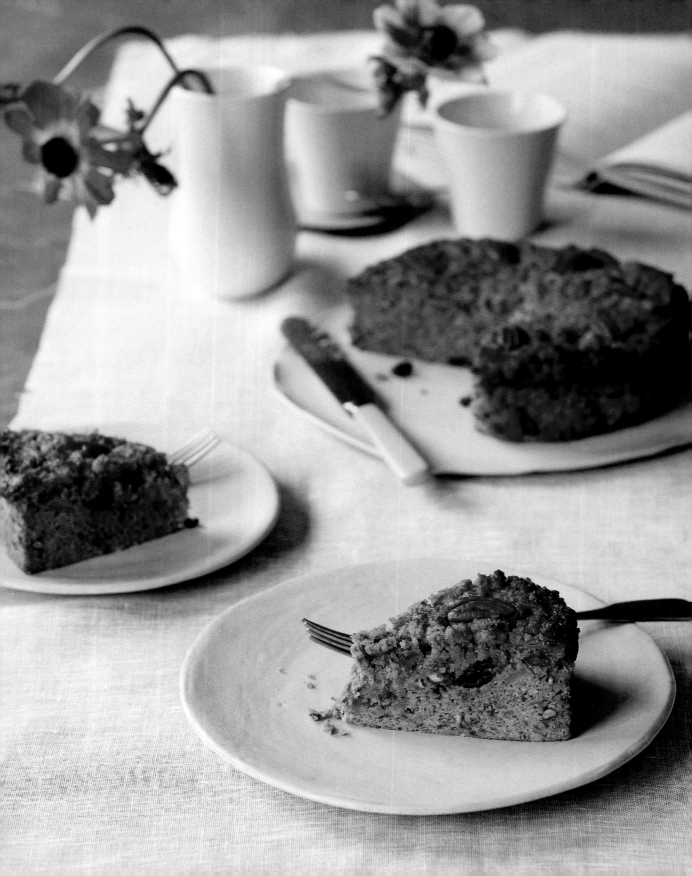

Carrot, pear, and ginger slice

Gingerbread and ginger cake were favorites of mine as a kid and that's before I knew how good ginger was for health! It's soothing and warming for the digestion and energizing, too. This recipe is made from carrots and nuts instead of flour, so is gluten-free, with a soft, light texture. **MAKES 12 SLICES**

1 Preheat the oven to 340°F [170°C]. Lightly oil a 7-in [23-cm] cake pan with coconut oil and line with parchment paper.

2 In one mixing bowl, stir the carrots and mashed pears. In another, sift all the dry ingredients. Drop the eggs and scant ½ cup (70 g) of the raisins into a food processor and blitz until smooth. Make a well in the dry ingredients and pour in the raisin mix, then the carrot mix, pecans, and remaining raisins. Fold in gently, then spoon into the pan. Top with the pecan halves.

3 Bake for 40 to 50 minutes, until a skewer inserted comes out clean. If the cake looks too golden during baking, cover loosely with parchment paper and return to the oven until cooked through.

a little coconut oil, for the pan

10½ oz [300 g] carrots, peeled and grated

2 ripe pears, peeled and mashed

1 tsp gluten-free baking powder

½ tsp baking soda

2¾ cups [250 g] ground almonds

⅓ cup [50 g] arrowroot

1½ tsp ground cinnamon

1 tsp ground ginger

4 extra-large eggs, lightly beaten

¾ cup [120 g] raisins

½ cup [75 g] pecans, coarsely chopped, plus pecan halves to decorate

Fig slice

I love these! Figs are fab as a mineral-booster and are highly alkalizing, too. **MAKES 25 SLICES**

1 Line a 13½-by-8-in [34-by-20-cm] brownie pan with parchment paper.

2 To make the base, combine the almonds, oats, coconut oil, dates, and vanilla in a food processor and blitz until it forms a sticky dough. Press it evenly into the prepared pan. Chill for one hour to firm up.

3 Preheat the oven to 350°F [180°C]. Soak the dried figs in hot water for 10 minutes. Drain them, pat dry, and mix with the cinnamon in a food processor until fairly smooth. Using a spatula, spread the filling on top of the base, then bake in the oven for 20 to 25 minutes, until the topping is sticky and golden.

4 Let cool for 10 minutes before cutting into squares. These can be eaten warm, but are also delicious cold.

FOR THE BASE

1⅔ cups [150 g] ground almonds

½ cup [50 g] rolled oats

2 Tbsp coconut oil

5 dates, pitted

1 tsp vanilla extract

FOR THE TOPPING

7 oz [200 g] dried figs

½ tsp ground cinnamon

Cashew soufflé with raspberries

Not just any old dessert, this is a heart-friendly, immune system, and sex-hormone boosting little puff in a ramekin! Cashews are high in selenium to help thyroid and immune function. Raspberries are a reminder of summer, and scientists now know that the metabolism in our fat cells can be increased by the phytonutrients they contain. The soufflé is also lactose-free and full of great fats and proteins for excellent mood, skin, and energy levels. Simply delicious … and dinner-party friendly, too.

SERVES 2

1⅓ cups [200 g] raw cashews

2 tsp raisins

15 raspberries, plus more to decorate

1 egg white

1 Preheat the oven to 400°F [200°C].

2 Place the cashews, raisins, raspberries, and ⅞ cup [200 ml] of filtered water in a blender (for best results, use a high-powered model such as a Vitamix) and blend until as smooth as possible.

3 Whisk the egg white until firm, then fold into the raspberry cashew cream. Pour the mixture into two ramekins; it should fill them to the top so you get a good rise.

4 Bake for 12 to 15 minutes. The soufflés will rise a little and turn light brown but remain soft in the center.

5 Serve hot, with a couple of raspberries dropped on top of each.

> I was told I couldn't make a soufflé without butter and milk … well, here it is!

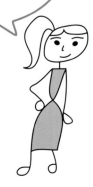

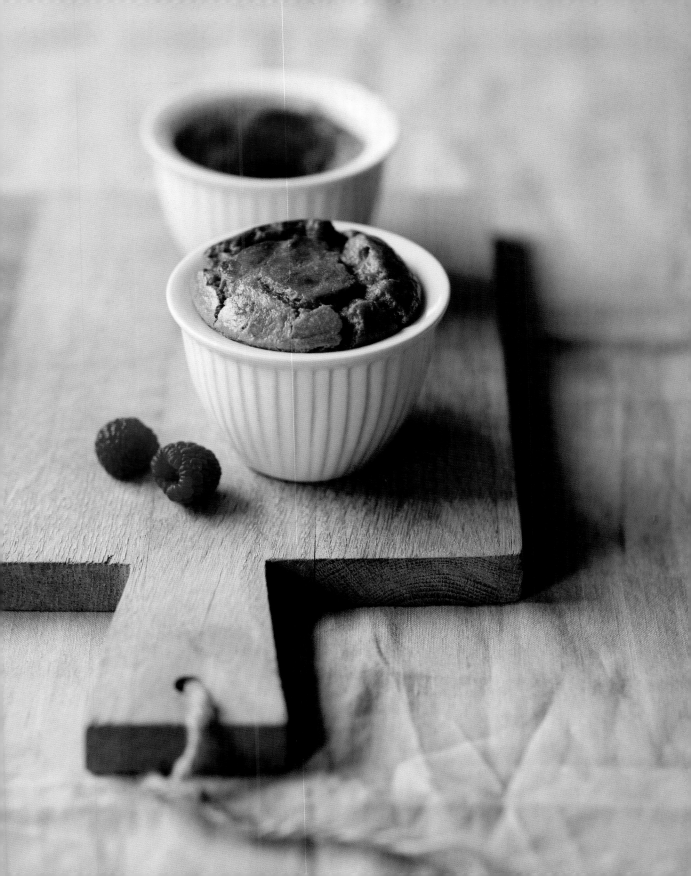

Apple and walnut cake

Walnut, apple, and raisin: What a yummy combination! And, beautifully, the protein in the walnuts "slows down" the fructose in the apple and raisins, so this cake won't cause a nasty blood sugar spike. This combination is alkalizing, antioxidant, and gives a good intake of magnesium and potassium. **ENOUGH FOR 12 SLICES**

1 Oil a 7-in [23-cm] cake pan and line the bottom with parchment paper.

2 Place the apples, lemon zest and juice, and raisins in a pan with 3 Tbsp of filtered water and simmer, covered, over low heat for 15 to 20 minutes, until slightly softened. Let cool. Preheat the oven to 350°F [180°C].

3 Whisk the eggs with an electric beater for five minutes, until thick and foamy. Fold in the ground almonds, baking powder, vanilla seeds, walnuts, and coconut oil until just combined, then briefly fold in the cooled stewed fruit mixture.

4 Transfer to the prepared pan and bake for 40 to 50 minutes, until golden and a skewer inserted into the center comes out clean. Let cool in the pan for 10 minutes before turning out and serving.

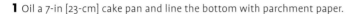

¼ cup [60 ml] coconut oil, melted, plus more for the pan

2 eating apples, peeled, cored, and coarsely chopped

finely grated zest and juice of ½ unwaxed lemon

1½ cups [250 g] raisins (or ¾ cup/ 125 g each raisins and chopped dried apricots, depending which you prefer)

5 extra-large eggs

2¾ cups [250 g] ground almonds

1½ tsp gluten-free baking powder

seeds of 1 vanilla bean

scant ½ cup [40 g] walnuts, coarsely chopped

Stellar Youthing Foods

What are the best youthing foods? Good question. A few points:

1 You can stack up your diet with pretty much any vegetable any time and know that youthing is happening. In other words, don't get caught up in the latest superfood superfad.

2 Some foods help with specific bodily processes such as detox, digestion, and alkalization, boost the immune system, or combat inflammation. In this section, I've chosen 45 nutrient-dense, new-normal foods to add to my original five—beet, garlic, lemon, red beans, turmeric—that I revealed in my *Eat Yourself Young* program, and targeted them to youthing processes they work on best. Try and eat a little more of these (and a little more often) for a great youthing start to the rest of your life. But be aware that many other foods offer youthing qualities. You can't go wrong if you follow point 1 above.

3 You'll notice there are no dairy products or meat in this list. I'd prefer you to get most of your protein from other sources: fish, nuts, seeds, veg, or beans. Not to say that all dairy or meat is nonyouthing: a little bit of red meat or a few spoons of plain, no-added-sugar yogurt with live cultures can be very healthful.

4 Most of these foods are used liberally in the recipes in this book. But just in case you want to ad lib, I've put in some "how to cook" tips.

AGAR (Digestion)
This plant-based "gelatin" is made from seaweed. It's fabulous for weight loss as it contains 80 percent fiber and makes you feel full, yet has negligible calories. It helps digestion, improves immunity, and creates a better youthing environment in the body.
How to cook: Use in desserts and custards. It sets as it cools.

ASPARAGUS (Detox)
Powerfully nutrient-dense, high not just in vitamins and minerals but also cancer-fighting compounds and amino acids that help detox at a cellular level, the Grail of antiaging. If you drink alcohol (moderately, of course!), asparagus can alleviate the after effects and protect hardworking liver cells.
How to cook: Serve as an appetizer or side, or chop into salad. Good as a soup.

AVOCADO (Alkalizing/Anti-Inflammatory)
Eat four times a week for younger-looking skin, hair, and nails. It has 25 vital nutrients/antioxidants including five anti-inflammatories, so it's a great all-round age-minimizer. It is 20 percent fat, but as this is healthy, cholesterol-reducing fat which helps suppress appetite, don't worry, just don't overeat it if you want to slim.
How to cook: Eat in guacamole and salads, use for creamy smoothies, ice creams, soups, and desserts.

BARLEY (Immune System/Digestion)
A body builder. It contains eight essential amino acids used for energy and repair in every cell. High in beta-glucan fiber (which helps reduce cholesterol) and potent antioxidants including a range of B-vitamins, it also helps PMT and insomnia: good sleep is the basis for regeneration.

How to cook: Use whole or pearl barley in risottos (nutty and delicious), soups, casseroles, and so on, or make barley water. Barley cakes and muffins have a sweet taste and chewy texture.

BEE POLLEN (Antioxidant/Anti-Inflammatory)
Useful as a natural sweetener to add to drinks, plus it has anti-inflammatory and antioxidant properties. It's pollen collected by bees mixed with nectar and bee saliva, and is high in protein, vitamins, and minerals (but avoid it if you're allergic to insect and bee stings).
How to cook: In nut milks, smoothies, sprinkled on breakfast cereals, or 1 tsp on its own for energy.

BUCKWHEAT (Antioxidant/Alkalizing)
A protein-rich seed that is wheat- and gluten-free. It has a nutty, almost malty flavor that I find delicious. It's dense in nutrients and antioxidants, essential amino acids, quercetin, rutin (youthing flavonoids), B-vitamins, and potassium. It's been shown to reduce cholesterol and protect against heart disease.
How to cook: Soak groats for 30 minutes, then make into an oatmeal or a rice substitute. Use in soups, risottos, and casseroles. The flour can be used in breads and pancakes.

CABBAGE (Detox)
A nutrient-dense cruciferous veg with high levels of glucosinolates that boost antioxidant uptake, help with detox, and protect against cell deterioration, so a good all-round youthing choice (as are broccoli, cauliflower, and other members of the cruciferous family).
How to cook: Raw (as coleslaw, in salads, juiced), fermented in sauerkraut, or only very lightly steamed, as active ingredients are lost through cooking.

CACAO NIBS (Antioxidant)
These are powerful antioxidants with a very high ORAC (Oxygen Radical Absorbance Capacity) value, which measures their ability to neutralize cell-damaging free radicals. They also lift your mood, raise energy, and solve chocolate cravings in a healthy way.

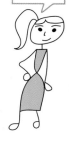

I often have 1 tsp of bee pollen when I need a quick lift; try it, it's sweet and delicious.

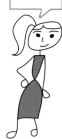

I spread half an avocado on sprouted bread toast for breakfast, for a super-youthing start to the day.

Stellar Youthing Foods

How to cook: Cacao nibs are very bitter so recipes often load in sugar. For the purposes of youthing, stay savory as the South Americans do and use cacao nibs in chili dishes and *mole* sauce. Or snack on them straight from the pack.

CARROT (Antioxidant)
I always say eat food that looks as close to its natural state as possible for genuine youthing. Carrots are a case in point: they contain high levels of beta-carotene and other antioxidants with protective powers against cancer, heart disease, high cholesterol, and even eyesight problems. But if the beta-carotene is extracted into little pills that you take instead of chomping carrots, all these benefits vanish.
How to cook: juice, eat raw or—better still—cooked (the nutrients are easier for the body to access), in soups, breads, cakes … Buy organic, or always peel them, as the skin can harbor pesticide residues.

CHAI TEA (Restorative)
I make this with cinnamon, cardamom, and star anise; you can add turmeric to increase its anti-inflammatory effects. It is soothing for the digestion, helps you kick caffeine, and is traditionally used as a mild anaesthetic and immune booster. Cinnamon stabilizes blood sugar and is known as an aphrodisiac.
How to cook: See page 45.

CHIA SEEDS (Digestive)
From a mint native to South America, traditionally eaten to boost energy. Nice amounts of anti-inflammatory omega-3 fatty acids, and antioxidants. They are great for gut health: high in fiber, and push things through speedily, which has a youthing knock-on for the immune system and the production of the happiness hormone: serotonin.
How to cook: Sprinkle on cereals, rice dishes, salads, or use to thicken sauces. Add a handful to smoothies and juices to help you absorb fat-soluble vitamins.

CHICKPEAS (Detox/Digestion/Antioxidant)
These delicious, buttery, nutty legumes are a great low-fat high-protein option. A good choice if you want to get leaner, as their starchy texture makes you feel full. They help reduce cholesterol and blood sugar and are high in iron and molybdenum, a mineral that helps detox the sulfites in processed foods and wine. With plentiful fiber and folic acid, they're youthing for the gut and encourage optimum cell functioning.
How to cook: Use dried (soak overnight, then drain and boil for two hours), canned (buy no-added salt), or as chickpea (gram) flour. Use in houmous, falafel, pies, curries, casseroles, and soups or on salads.

CIDER VINEGAR (Alkalizing)
This acid, when metabolized, pushes the body to alkalinity and helps joint pain, fatigue, dull hair, dry skin, bone health, and other overacidity issues. It reduces blood sugar and cholesterol and also weight, as it makes you feel full. Use unpasteurized vinegar from health food stores, it's more youthing.
How to cook: Use in salad dressings, or add a dash to hot pots. I drink 1 Tbsp in warm water before meals if I'm feeling a little acidic, or need help digesting …

COCONUT MILK (Alkalizing)
This is so hip, and for the right reasons. It's highly alkalizing, a good source of minerals (potassium, manganese, molybdenum, calcium, magnesium, and zinc), and medium-chain fats that fight bacteria and fungi, which is why upping your intake can help with candida (see page 28). It's high in calories though, so don't go bonkers.
How to cook: Ideally see page 46 to make it, or you can buy cans of whole milk, not the low-fat version (from which the "good" fats have been removed). Use wherever you would milk, on cereal, in curries, soup, baking (pancakes, scones, cakes), in ice creams, smoothies, and so on. It brings a lovely velvety richness to dishes.

CUCUMBER (Alkalizing)
Nothing beats cucumber for dewy skin and I love it for youthing generally. It's high in silica, which helps keep connective tissue healthy (the muscles, ligaments, tendons,

cartilage and bone that hold you together). Plus it's low-cal, so great for munchies.
How to cook: It is better raw, for the crunchiness. Use in juices, salads, and cold soups. Buy organic, or else the skin is waxed or has pesticide residues and that's the bit that contains the most silica.

CURRANTS, BLACK AND RED
(Anti-Inflammatory/Antioxidant)
Yes, they have a short summer window but currants are superrich in GLA (gamma-linolenic acid) which is very, very good for skin (including difficult-to-treat conditions such as eczema). An anti-inflammatory that is also high in antioxidants, these are all-round youthing and taste intensely gorgeous.
How to cook: Eat raw with coconut cream or add to ice cream. Poach to make into a coulis (strain it, to seed, if you prefer) to pour over cereals or fruit desserts. Try frozen when fresh are not available.

DAIKON (Detox/Digestion)
Or "mooli": This is a radish that looks like a fat white carrot. It has digestive enzymes similar to those in humans, so is said to help with digestion of fat and protein. It's high in vitamin C, folic acid, and potassium, which is

great for detox as it can help keep cells at their optimum youthing electrolyte balance (5:1 potassium to sodium).
How to cook: Steam or roast, but raw (grated on salads, or as a side) is best for enzyme uptake. I juice them with other veg for a sharp, radishy detox.

EDAMAME BEANS (Digestion)
These young soybeans in the pod provide a complete protein, so are wonderful for vegetarians and vegans. Plus they are full of vitamins B, C, K, and high in fiber. All of which makes them a very healthy and youthing option, unless they are drenched in salt, as is often the case in sushi and snack bars.
How to cook: Simmer for five minutes, then eat as a snack or on salads.

HEMP SEEDS (Anti-Inflammatory/Antioxidant)
Not just for hippies! High in omega-3s (that reduce inflammation, cholesterol, and cardiac risk); high in digestible protein (good for raising energy levels); great for older, dry, and problem skins. Plus they contain many of the finest antioxidant vitamins and minerals for optimum youthing.
How to cook: Buy unhulled seeds to make into milk (see page 46); they are more expensive, but you can add them to smoothies, sprinkle on cereals, in casseroles, and so on. You can also buy hemp oil (see page 11) as a neat way to get all of hemp's youthing benefits …

HORSERADISH (Digestion/Detox)
I'm a huge fan of this, I eat it with salmon and adore the punch of horseradish mash. Antioxidant (especially high in vitamin C) and anti-inflammatory. It's also a good detoxer; by stimulating bile it helps digest fats and eliminate cholesterol and other wastes. (But grate it in a well-ventilated room!)
How to cook: Use raw for maximum pungency. Grate and mix with plain yogurt, cider vinegar, or grated apple as a sauce for beans or fish. To make horseradish mash, grate 1 Tbsp into mashed potatoes, celeriac, or beet. Store in the refrigerator.

KALE (Alkalizing/Detox)
A nutritional powerhouse, probably the most palatable way to get a big shot of calcium in a low-cal way (though parsley, garlic, and dandelion leaves are up there …). High in cancer-fighting sulforaphane and carotenes, it also helps the regeneration and repair of your cells: very youthing!
How to cook: Juice, steam, steam-fry; add to soups, casseroles, mash (to make colcannon), or make "Cheesy" kale chips (see page 75).

KIWI (Antioxidant/Immune-Boosting)
A good little youthing helper: full of vitamin C, E, potassium, magnesium, and dietary fiber. It's a very low-sugar fruit so is great in the morning with yogurt or nuts and seeds. Or if you fancy a sweet snack that won't shoot your blood levels sky high, this is it.
How to cook: Eat raw, juice, in tarts.

LICORICE ROOT (Restorative)
The best sugar-free treat. Around 50 times sweeter than sugar, but doesn't rot your teeth, in fact it may protect them. It helps you cope with stress (as an adrenal and liver tonic), is anti-inflammatory, and can protect against ulcers. (Don't have more than two sticks or teas a week and, if you have high blood pressure, avoid it.)
How to cook: Chew a stick or make tea (steep in boiled water for five minutes).

MACKEREL (Anti-Inflammatory)
Like all oily fish (salmon, sardines, herring), high in omega-3 fatty acids, which help reduce cholesterol, protect against heart disease, and cancer and ease joint pain and arthritis (the anti-inflammatory effect). Good for depression and memory; high in vitamin D that fights dementia.
How to cook: Broil or bake with tart or anise flavors: try gooseberry or fennel.

MAPLE SYRUP
Drilled from a hole in the maple tree. It's high in manganese and zinc and contains calcium, potassium, and iron. It's a whole lot better than sugar, but also sweet: eat with caution.

MINT (Digestion)
The powerful aroma is a dead giveaway: those pungent oils do great things for your stomach, soothe bloating and inflammation, relax muscles, and help your digestion function at its youthing best. Plus it tastes divine, too.
How to cook: Raw in salads (including fruit salads), tabbouleh, in any cooked veg dish, as mint tea, or in ice cream.

MUSHROOMS: SHIITAKE AND MAITAKE (Immune-Boosting)
Go for these over regular 'shrooms: they offer a rejuvenating boost. They reduce cholesterol, while a compound called lentinan powers immunity and helps fight infection and disease. Maitake are hard to find (you might have to buy dried) but contain beta-glucans that are immune-boosting and destroy malignant cells while protecting healthy ones.
How to cook: Add to soups, casseroles, savory dishes, and omelets.

NIGELLA SEEDS (Anti-Inflammatory/Detox/Digestive/Antioxidant)
Hot and peppery, they make everything taste of India! They are widely used as a liver and kidney detoxer, are anti-inflammatory, antifungal, antibacterial (so soothing for the gut), anticancer, and can help to reduce blood pressure. They are antioxidant, too: high in vitamin C and minerals (especially iron and calcium). These are powerful things, so check with your doctor before using if you are on any anticancer, kidney, or liver medication.
How to cook: Use 1 tsp in a spice mix for fish, meat, or veg dishes; grind, and add to salad dressings or rice. Roast and eat (if you're feeling brave) as a snack.

NUTMEG (Anti-Inflammatory)
Good sleep is regenerative and youth-enhancing and, if you find it hard to get your nightly shift, ¼ tsp nutmeg in warm nut milk a few hours before bed may help. Nutmeg is anti-inflammatory and traditionally has also been used to lift mood and ease gas.
How to cook: Buy whole and grate just before you need it. Also good in nut and seed milks, desserts, baked goods, and savory dishes.

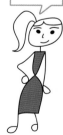

I chew licorice when I want a bit of sweet, or add it to mint tea; it's antibacterial so good for gums and gum health.

Stellar Youthing Foods

NUTS (Anti-Inflammatory)
Love 'em! That's why I gave them a whole section (see page 12).

OCTOPUS/SQUID (Antioxidant/Anti-Inflammatory)
People eat these in restaurants, but won't dish them up at home. Big mistake! Power-packed nutritionally and easy to cook (see page 69), high in vitamins (including hard-to-get B-12), minerals, and antioxidants including taurine (which reduces blood pressure and cholesterol). A good source of omega-3 fatty acids—especially DHA which is great for the brain, memory, and concentration—and, because it is short-lived, contains fewer toxins than many fish and seafoods.

OILS (Anti-Inflammatory)
We need healthy fats and my favorites are avocado, coconut, hemp, olive, and pumpkin seed oils. They are anti-inflammatory, high in omega fatty acids, antioxidant, high in vitamins and minerals, and protein-dense. They reduce cholesterol, help rejuvenate skin, hair and nails, fuel the metabolism, help us absorb fat-soluble vitamins ... and feed our brains! The best nutrients and flavors are in virgin, first cold-pressed oils.
How to use: See page 10–11.

PARSNIP (Digestion)
Naturally high in sugars, parsnip is very high in soluble and insoluble fiber, which reduces blood cholesterol and helps gut function. It also contains minerals—especially phosphorus and potassium—the latter counteracts an oversodium-ized life and promotes a youthing electrolyte balance in the body.
How to cook: Juice with other veg (it adds sweet creaminess); roast; mash with rutabaga or celeriac; use in soup.

PESTO (Alkalizing/Antioxidant)
Basically any strong-tasting green veg blended with garlic, olive oil, and nuts, this is very youthing: antioxidant, alkalizing, with healthy monounsaturated fats, and cholesterol-reducing (because of the garlic).
How to cook: Make with basil, arugula, parsley,

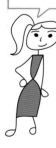

I notice my hair is better when I eat quinoa regularly. I put it down to the lysine, an amino acid linked to tissue growth and repair.

nettle (steam young spring leaves for two minutes first), or watercress or cauliflower leaves, or any mixture that appeals.

PINTO BEANS (Antioxidant/Digestion)
Any beans are good beans (except canned baked beans, or any with added sugar or salt) but pinto beans are beautiful, too. Pinkish when cooked and with a creamy flavor, they have all the highlights of beans (high in protein, nutrients, and antioxidants, low in fat) and are exceptionally high in fiber, which gives the digestion a workout.
How to cook: Use dried or canned (no-sugar, no-salt varieties) to make dips, soups, casseroles, salads, and burgers.

POMEGRANATE (Anti-Inflammatory/Immune Booster)
I love fresh pomegranate (forget the manufactured juice) for its flavor and "popping" texture. Crunchy, tangy, bittersweet, it acts as an anti-inflammatory and artery-declogger, and also protects against heart disease and viral infections.
How to cook: Use it in salads, in sauces with meat, as a relish, in ice cream ...

QUINOA (Digestion/Restorative)
The "gold of the Incas," a great protein source for the gluten- and wheat-free. I recommend it for youthing as it's a seed not a grain and contains all the essential amino acids, plus a healthy dose of vitamins, minerals, and fiber. It's high in vitamin B2 that is vital for energy metabolism; and iron and potassium, which help every cell function at its youthing best.
How to cook: Cook on its own or chuck, raw, into soups and casseroles (it's nutritionally excellent with beans). In fact it is super-versatile: I love it with chopped fruit and seeds for breakfast, cold in a salad, or drizzled with olive oil and pepper for supper. You can also sprout it. Try quinoa flour when baking.

RADISH (Detox/Digestion)
Underrated and underused in the West, radishes are fabulous detoxers; if ever you feel like an inner cleanse, grab a radish and munch! One of the cruciferous vegetables,

*** *** ***

YOU EAT HEALTHILY BUT WANT TO LOSE WEIGHT?
Simple: Limit the sweetness in your life
People gorge on youthing foods, thinking they are doing right by their body. But some are high in calories and sugars, so you need to use a bit of smart thinking if you want to lose weight as well. Try these supersimple guidelines for one month and just see how much leaner and younger you feel:

Avoid completely
Dried fruits, fruit juice, alcohol, maple and other syrups, agave nectar, sweeteners of any kind, cow's, goat, and sheep dairy, wheat, and grains (because they can irritate the gut).

Eat sparingly
Nuts, seeds, fish, red and white meats, fruit (maximum two pieces a day).

Eat lots of
Agar (makes you feel full); asparagus; vegetable proteins such as chickpeas, edamame, pea protein, hemp, sprouted foods, legumes, pinto and other beans, quinoa; chia seeds; daikon, kale, radishes; seaweed; veg and herb medleys (carrots, cabbage, cucumber, parsley, watercress, you name it).

*** *** ***

they have that trademark sulfurous zesty tang: it's these chemicals that help improve digestion (and youthing). They are low-cal, high-fiber, and anti-inflammatory.
How to cook: Delicious raw in salads, or dipped in nutritional yeast. Steam radishes with other veg (beet, carrots, sweet potatoes); they add a sharp antidote to any sweetness. Or slice thinly and use in stir-fries.

SEA VEGETABLES (Restorative)
Or seaweed in all its guises from arame and dulse to kelp, kombi, nori, samphire, and wakame, a youthing must-eat a couple

of times a week. The most mineral-dense food on earth, it is especially rich in iodine, which helps produce the thyroid hormones which affect metabolism, mood, weight, and energy. It's thought to help prevent estrogen-dependent cancers, is anti-inflammatory; and helps the body cope with stress (and menopausal symptoms …). Just one thing to be wary of: it may aggravate acne flare-ups.

How to cook: With a fantastic natural salty flavor, it usually comes dried, though you can get fresh samphire for a short summer season: steam or eat raw in salads. Use dried seaweed flakes or ground nori as a seasoning, sprinkle over egg dishes, salads, or add to juices. You can also soak dried sea veg for 30 minutes before using in Japanese appetizers or broth: be adventurous!

SPROUTED FOODS (Restorative)

You can sprout any seeds, beans, or grains … but why would you? Simple: it makes food more nutrient-dense and digestible and thus more youthing. Each seed is a life force: it contains all it needs to grow into a plant. Soaking and sprouting kicks off that growth process: enzymes break down the seed's toxic defenses and create protein, fiber, minerals, and vitamins, which we then eat.

How to sprout and cook: Use a seed sprouter or large glass jar. Rinse your seeds thoroughly, then soak in water for 12 to 24 hours. Discard any floaters. Pour off the water and rinse again. Lay them out in the seed sprouter or jar turned on its side, rinsing once or twice a day. They are ready to eat when they reach about ¼ in (5 mm) (in three or four days). Eat raw but not by the handful, as they can contain toxins. Cook in stir-fries, or steam as a side.

SQUASH AND SWEET POTATOES

(Antioxidant/Anti-Inflammatory)
High in protective carotenes and anti-inflammatory, these help regulate blood sugar, and are youthing for skin and muscles.

How to cook: Roast to make into soups, add (chopped) to casseroles, curries, and risottos. Mash. Spaghetti squash can be baked, then used instead of spaghetti.

TOMATO (Antioxidant/Anti-Inflammatory)
The most versatile vegetable (or fruit, depending on how pedantic you are). Eat ripe and red as they then contain more lycopene, an antioxidant that protects against cell deterioration and keeps you looking and feeling younger.

How to cook: Raw, paste, canned, all are good (though I am not wild about the sugar and additives in ketchup or some cans, so avoid them). Eat raw in salads. Cook in pizzas or make tomato sauce.

VANILLA (Antioxidant/Restorative)
It adds a fabulous richness of flavor to sweet dishes, helps reduce anxiety and stress, lifts the spirits, and regulates metabolism … all very youthing! Plus it is extremely high on the ORAC (Oxygen Radical Absorbance Capacity) scale, which measures how powerfully antioxidants slow the effects of age-related degeneration and disease.

How to cook: Scrape the seeds from beans and use to flavor teas, juices, ice cream, custards, sauces, desserts, and so on. For a counterintuitive taste experience, try grinding a little black pepper into a vanilla custard, it's yummy.

WATERCRESS (Alkalizing/Detox)
Does this need any introduction as a superfood? It's low-cal yet busting with vitamins, minerals, and antioxidants and contains sulfurophanes which help cells defend themselves from carcinogens and degeneration. Its deep green color and peppery taste are a giveaway that it's alkalizing, detoxing, and generally good for head-to-toe youthing.

How to cook: Eat raw in salads; juice; make into a tea (infuse for 10 minutes); for soup or pesto; add to mash or tarts.

WHEATGRASS (Alkalizing/Detox)
This makes your skin, hair, nails, and eyes shine. High in chlorophyll, vitamins A, B-12, and E and many minerals, it's a powerful detoxifier and alkalizer, but hold your nose as you drink it. The more you need it, the more your liver wants to make you vomit!

EAT FERMENTED FOR A HAPPY GUT
Miso, sauerkraut, kefir, kimchi, tempeh … most cultures around the world sussed out centuries ago that fermenting foods made them easier to digest and more nutritious, too.

Fermenting breaks down carbs and, as a side effect, produces lovely levels of enzymes and probiotics that help your gut stay healthy and digest food better. When your gut flora is in good shape, your immune system works well, you absorb the minerals and vitamins you need and your body and mind function at their best.

Some people say that eating fermented foods helps improve skin, mood, energy, and their zest for life … perhaps because, in a healthy gut, candida, and the fatigue and depression it causes are kept at bay.

Fermented foods are intense taste bombs, so eat with other dishes for a full-on flavor experience. Little and often is my advice: add 1 Tbsp of miso to casseroles, eat sauerkraut (best to make your own), or have a spoonful of kefir on your breakfast cereal every now and then

---

How to cook: Juice it fresh, or sprinkle the powder on soups and savory dishes.

YEAST, NUTRITIONAL (Restorative)
This has a fabulous nutty, cheesy flavor and is an excellent source of protein for vegans and vegetarians. Make sure you buy the yeast fortified with vitamin B-12: it contains all the essential amino acids and B-complex vitamins you need for a robust nervous system and healthy metabolism. Low in fat and salt, it's a youthing winner.

How to cook: Sprinkle over salads, crudités, and popcorn, use in soups, juices, and casseroles and to make vegan "cheese" (see page 81).

Fresh samphire steamed for two or three minutes, served with sliced summer-ripe tomatoes and black olives and drizzled with olive oil, is a fantastic side with white fish.

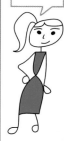

I eat a lot of sprouted bread which I always buy. One day I intend to go all out and make it myself and then I will write about it!

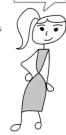

Index

Acknowledgments

My really heartfelt thanks goes out to my husband Richard, my mother Eva Peyton-Jones and my stepchildren Thomas and Hamish, who have been so supportive and understanding throughout this long (and at times tedious) process. I am lucky to have a rather large immediate family and my sisters are an amazing sisterhood, with endless time, ears, and encouragement; thank you thank you, they may become the feature of my next book! My ageless and elegant Aunt Peggy is, as ever, in the background of all my endeavors.

I would like to thank Jane for helping me with my words and the whole team at Quadrille who made this all possible.

Publishing Director: Sarah Lavelle
Creative Director: Helen Lewis
Project Editor: Lucy Bannell
Art Direction and Design: Katherine Keeble
Photography: Yuki Sugiura
Illustration: Katherine Keeble
Co-writer: Jane Phillimore
Recipe developers and home economists:
Emily Jonzen and Cyntra Hinde
Food stylist: Camilla Baynham
Props stylist: Cynthia Inions
Production: Vincent Smith, Tom Moore

First published in 2015 by
Quadrille Publishing Limited
Pentagon House
52–54 Southwark Street
London SE1 1UN
www.quadrille.com

Quadrille is an imprint of Hardie Grant
www.hardiegrant.com.au

Reprinted in 2016
10 9 8 7 6 5 4 3 2

Text © 2015 Elizabeth Peyton-Jones
Photography © 2015 Yuki Sugiura
Design and layout © 2015 Quadrille
Publishing Limited

Cataloguing in Publication Data: a catalogue record for this book is available from the British Library.

ISBN: 978 184949 679 7

Printed in China